Emergency Admissions:
A journey in the right direction?

A report of the National Confidential Enquiry into Patient Outcome and Death (2007)

Compiled by:

I C Martin LLM FRCS FDSRCS
Lead Clinical Co-ordinator

D G Mason FFARCS
Clinical Co-ordinator

J Stewart FRCP LLM
Clinical Co-ordinator

M Mason PhD
Chief Executive

N C E Smith BSc PhD
Clinical Researcher

K Gill BSc
Research Assistant

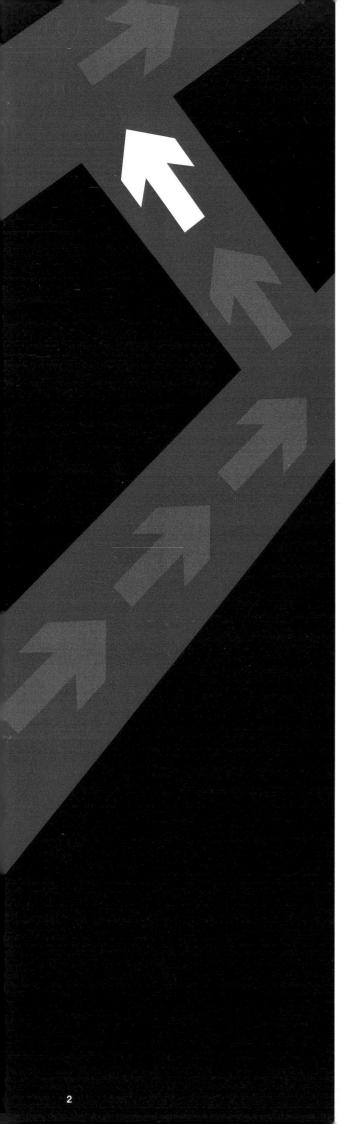

Contents

Acknowledgements

This is the twentieth report published by NCEPOD and, as always, could not have been achieved without the support of a wide range of individuals and organisations. Our particular thanks go to:

The Expert Group who advised NCEPOD:

Dr Chris Roseveare
Consultant Physician

Ms Elaine Cole
Senior Sister, Emergency Medicine

Mr James Halsey
Patient and Carer Network,
Royal College of Physicians (London)

Professor Matthew Cooke
Professor of Emergency Medicine

Mr Paul Hurst
Consultant Surgeon

Dr Roop Kishen
Consultant in Intensive Care Medicine & Anaesthesia

Professor Terry Wardle
Consultant Gastroenterologist

Ms Tanya Reynolds
Nurse

Ms Joanna Fisher
Nurse

Professor Ian Gilmore
Consultant Physician and Gastroenterologist

Dr Michael Bacon
Consultant Physician

Mr Richard Novell
Consultant Surgeon

Mr Peter Dawson
Consultant Surgeon

Dr Andrew Volans
Consultant in Emergency Medicine

Dr Simon Carley
Consultant in Emergency Medicine

The Advisors who reviewed the cases:

Dr Alastair Douglas
Consultant Physician in Nephrology and Acute Medicine

Miss Catherine Davies
Nurse Consultant, Critical Care

Dr David Perks
Medical Service Head, Anaesthetics,
Critical Care and Theatres

Dr David Vickery
Consultant in Emergency Medicine

Dr George Noble
Consultant Physician

Dr Hugh Bradby
Consultant Gastroenterologist

Ms Mandy Williams
Senior Sister

Mrs Marilyn Gagg
Ward Manager

Dr Ruth Green
Consultant Respiratory and General Physician

Dr Simon Chapman
Specialist Registrar in Accident and Emergency

Dr Chris Maimaris
Emergency Medicine Consultant

Mr Daniel Wolstenholme
Research Development Advisor

Dr Daren Forward
Specialist Registrar in Trauma and Orthopaedic Surgery

Mr David Redfern
Consultant Trauma & Orthopaedic Surgeon

Mr John Abercrombie
Consultant Colorectal Surgeon

Dr Ken Lowry
Consultant in Intensive Care Medicine

Dr Kevin Kiff
Consultant Anaesthesia & Intensive Care Medicine

Mr Mark Radford
Consultant Nurse

Mr Nigel Andrews
Consultant General and Gastroenterological Surgeon

Mr Tim Lees
Consultant Vascular Surgeon

Acknowledgements

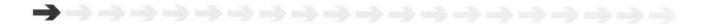

The organisations that provided funding to cover the cost of this study:

National Patient Safety Agency

Department of Health, Social Services and Public Safety (Northern Ireland)

Aspen Healthcare

Benenden Hospital

BMI Healthcare

BUPA

Capio Group

Covenant Healthcare

Cromwell Hospital

Isle of Man Health and Social Security Department

Fairfield Independent Hospital

HCA International

Horder Centre

Hospital Management Trust

Hospital of St John and St Elizabeth

King Edward VII Hospital

King Edward VIIs Hospital Sister Agnes

London Clinic

McIndoe Surgical Centre

Mount Alvernia Hospital

Netcare Healthcare

New Victoria Hospital

North Wales Medical Centre

Nuffield Hospitals

Orchard Hospital

St Anthony's Hospital

St Joseph's Hospital

Spencer Wing,
Queen Elizabeth the Queen Mother Hospital

States of Guernsey, Health and Social Services

States of Jersey, Health and Social Services

Ulster Independent Clinic

The professional organisations that support our work and who constitute our Steering Group:

Association of Anaesthetists of Great Britain and Ireland

Association of Surgeons of Great Britain and Ireland

Coroners' Society of England and Wales

Faculty of Dental Surgery of the Royal College of Surgeons of England

Faculty of Public Health of the Royal College of Physicians of the UK

Institute of Healthcare Management

Royal College of Anaesthetists

Royal College of Child Health and Paediatrics

Royal College of General Practitioners

Royal College of Nursing

Royal College of Obstetricians and Gynaecologists

Royal College of Ophthalmologists

Royal College of Pathologists

Royal College of Physicians of London

Royal College of Radiologists

Royal College of Surgeons of England

The authors and Trustees of NCEPOD would particularly like to thank the NCEPOD staff for their hard work in collecting and analysing the data for this study:

Robert Alleway, Sabah Begg, Philip Brown, Heather Cooper, Sidhaarth Gobin, Clare Holtby, Dolores Jarman, Viki Pepper, Saba Raza, and Donna Weyman.

In addition we thank our scientific advisors *Dr Martin Utley* and *Professor Steve Gallivan* for all their assistance.

Furthermore thanks go to all the NCEPOD Local Reporters who identified cases for this study, and to all the clinicians that completed the questionnaires.

Disclaimer

This work was undertaken by NCEPOD, which received funding for this report from the National Patient Safety Agency. The views expressed in this publication are those of the authors and not necessarily those of the Agency.

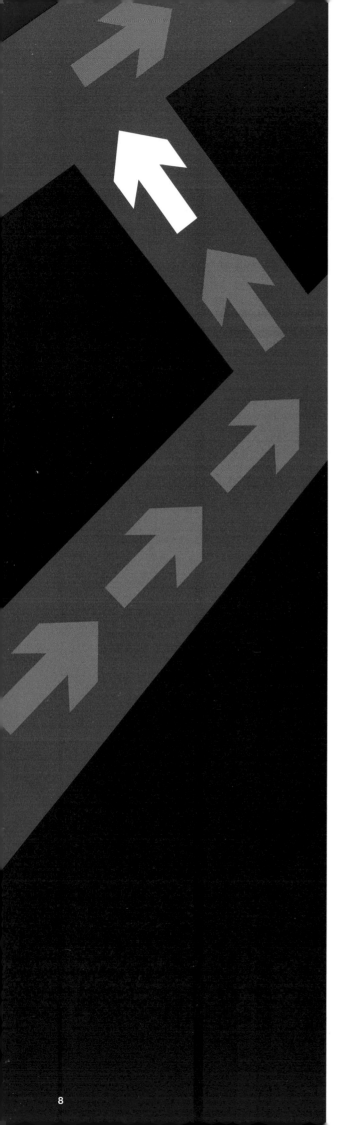

Foreword

At a funeral recently I listened as a man talked of the death of his wife, the mother of three children still finding their feet in the adult world. She had died of lung cancer taking 18 months on her way from diagnosis to death. "Well, I'm thankful it was cancer" he said. His words cut through the sadness and impressed upon me something I had never quite thought through before. Thankful? Cancer? Yes. There had been time – time to talk, think, reminisce, plan and time for both of them at each stage to choose what happened next. People sent into hospital for emergency admission usually have little time for choice, nor the control, autonomy and self determination that go with it.

Time is critical in acute illness. In the case of catastrophic cardiovascular events such as heart attack, pulmonary embolism, stroke or internal bleeding, what happens next might mean the difference between life and death - time measured in hours and minutes. "Time is heart muscle" we say, to prompt early diagnosis and treatment in heart attacks. What is done or not done in those first few hours determines not only whether the patient will survive, but how quickly and completely health and independence might be restored.

Medicine, as we know it now, offers opportunities to change the course of events in acute illness in ways undreamt of when I first encountered emergency admissions as a clinical medical student in 1967. Then, if a patient presented with an acute coronary event we more or less sat it out with some supportive care in the form of morphine and oxygen. Now, intravenous nitrates, a confident diagnosis by detection of troponin release, intravenous thrombolysis, and access to 24 hour catheter laboratories for imaging and percutaneous interventions allow us to do something really effective to alter the course of events. Similarly, management of cardiac arrhythmia, pulmonary embolism, and gastrointestinal bleeding have been transformed by sophisticated monitoring and measurement, imaging and therapeutic interventions. These save lives but not only that - they preserve the function of the vital organs that will determine future health.

So that is what is now possible and it has developed over forty years spent caring for patients many of whom, in my own life's work, arrived in hospital as acute admissions with diseases affecting their lungs and cardiovascular systems. But can this care be delivered? Is it being delivered? The theoretical possibility of saving life and restoring health amounts to little if these measures cannot be implemented widely and promptly. The practitioners have to have the resources to be able to deliver, and then to get it right. Reducing the clotting of blood by thrombolysis saves a life if the life is threatened by intra-coronary thrombus or pulmonary embolism, but it does the patient no favour if the problem is a leaking aneurysm or an internal bleed. It is not just about technology – it is as much about people with skills, training, judgement, and reflection, engaged in closely co-ordinated team work. Can we, and do we, deliver that?

As the technology has changed so have the practitioners. We might look back to the golden days of yore when the hospitals were staffed day and night by highly competent, experienced and battle hardened senior registrars. We saw patients in the casualty department and we took care of them whether in the intensive care unit or the operating theatres, day and night. And there was built into it an inevitable continuity of care, for the same doctors had done the clinics, ward rounds and operating yesterday and would do them again tomorrow. Well, reminisce if you wish, but those days are gone and will not come back, in part because they were not in reality that golden. Modern care demands expertise in acute care, diagnosis, resuscitation and treatment. It demands

specialists with technical expertise to obtain and read the sophisticated echo, CT and MRI images, to interpret the diagnostic tests, and to drive the kit – if interventions are to succeed and harm is to be avoided. It is not a single talented omnipotent individual but a process staffed by many people. What are the failings and how could they be addressed? That is the area of enquiry of the Emergency Admissions study.

Can NCEPOD's methods capture all the facets of care that might favourably or adversely influence the outcome for an individual patient? Well it has not been easy. We targeted patient groups (those that died or remained in intensive care) that were likely to test the system and to reveal shortcomings. Data have been retrieved from clinical records. We can never and do not attempt to say whether the outcome for the patient would certainly have been different if some other course of action had been taken; a decision had been made more promptly; another facility had been available; a missed clinical clue had been acted upon; or different people had done different things in a different way. Whilst a prospective study with a control group works to measure the effect of one intervention compared with another (as in a controlled trial) the reality of the emergency admission is that there is an unending cycle of evaluation, diagnosis and intervention rendering it inaccessible to formal hypothesis testing. That said, we constantly explore within NCEPOD more objective ways of drawing inferences and reaching conclusions to augment the human judgements drawn from the lifetimes' experience of our expert advisors about what is a very human process.

The most human of all factors is the humanity of the patient. The very nature of the emergency takes from them what they might want most in their illness – to understand what is going on, to be given explanations and to be able to retain some choice, some control, and

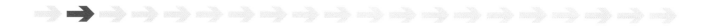

some vestige of self determination. The experience of a patient admitted in an emergency can be as bewildering as that experienced by Kafka's characters – others appear to take control and make major decisions which affect their very survival and yet the patient is ill equipped and in no position to know how or why these people act. And so I return to the image of the man telling the story of the loss of his wife with cancer. He had seen friends and family die before: a young brother in law killed outright, hit by a speeding car; the children's grandmother taken by a stroke and dead in hours. No time. Foreshortening of time is the nature of the emergency. The pressure to make decisions and to act on them leaves little time to explain – and the reality is that the hospital team do not themselves always know what is going on, and what might happen next, and what should be done then. In emergency care, diagnoses and plans are provisional and as events unfold, must change. How do we explain that to the patient and to the family?

In the care of Emergency Admissions, explanations have to be given after the event. Sometimes it is to explain how a happy outcome was achieved, an inevitable death was peaceful and dignified, but sometimes it is to express sorrow and regret after a death. Questions might include: "Might things have gone better if you had acted sooner?" "Would she be still alive if there had been an intensive care bed?" "Why did his last hours have to be spent on a trolley moving from ward to ward?" In a sense the questions that the family might ask are questions the study posed. While reading this report, it should be noted that we deliberately sampled patients on the basis of specifically weighted outcomes selected to reveal where the system might have been stressed to breaking point;

we do not claim to have evaluated the overall standard of the service. Although inadequacies in organisational or clinical care appear small when individual components are considered, only 61.6% of patients in the groups sampled in this study received an overall standard of care considered by our advisors to be consistent with good practice. There were remediable factors, either clinical or organisational, in the standard of care received by the remaining 34.8% of these patients. Not all of these will have affected the outcome but all of them represent shortcomings of the service provided to very ill people.

Professor T. Treasure
Chairman

Introduction

Emergency admissions to hospital are, by definition, unpredictable and unexpected in the individual case, even where the system has been properly set up to cater for them. Such admissions account for approximately one third of all admissions and in 2004-2005 increased by 6.5% on the previous year to 4.43 million[1].

The volume and unpredictability of these admissions is a significant part of the health service. Consequently, there has been considerable interest within both governmental and non-governmental organisations as to how to manage these demands [2-6]. Previous reports have concentrated on the initial care of patients: primarily on access to emergency care and the organisational and clinical management of emergency admissions. Moreover, a national audit of emergency medical admissions reported that the most significant problems at admission were sub-optimal involvement of consultants in acute care and the fact that the admitting specialty is frequently inappropriate to the patient's condition[7]. While the first response on admission is certainly an important point of focus, it is equally important to look at the organisation of subsequent care. To date, very little work has been reported in this area.

In this study, NCEPOD has assessed organisational and clinical aspects of both the immediate and ongoing care of patients admitted as emergencies. The report highlights remediable factors in existing care pathways, particularly the appropriateness, timeliness and frequency of investigations and reviews, the experience of staff and the availability of results, protocols and procedures.

NCEPOD deliberately sampled an acutely ill group of patients because remediable factors in their care are likely to be more obvious, giving insights into the inherent problems and inefficiencies within the acute sector.

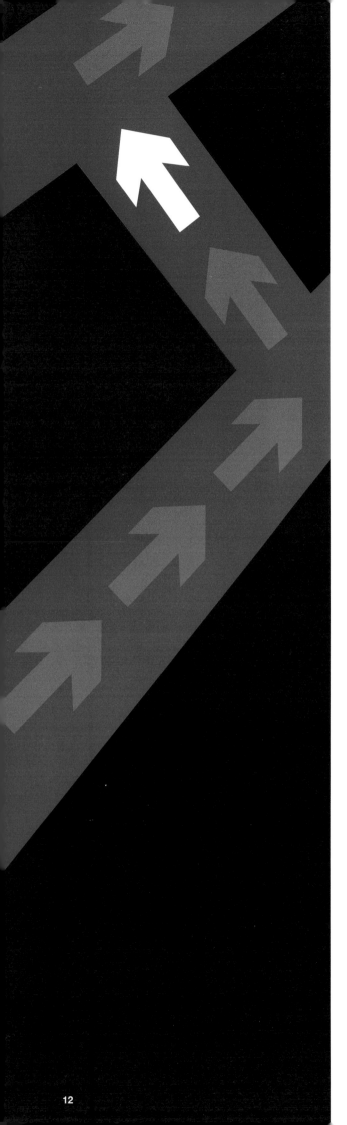

Overview of findings

Patients admitted as an emergency can be amongst the sickest that are cared for in hospital. This report highlights the need for early decision making by doctors with the most appropriate skills and knowledge based on the clinical needs of the patient. Clinicians and managers should review current arrangements for the delivery of care to this group of patients.

- 34.8% of patients had remediable factors identified in their clinical and/or organisational standard of care received. Not all of these would have affected their outcome but all represent shortcomings of the service provided to very ill people.

- 7.1% of cases had an initial assessment that was assessed, by the advisors, as poor or unacceptable. Patients admitted as an emergency should be seen initially by a doctor with the necessary skills and knowledge to make a competent clinical assessment, devise a differential diagnosis and appropriate management plan. At the very least, this doctor should have the first of these competencies and have immediate access to a more senior doctor who can formulate the latter two requirements. Furthermore, there were examples within this study of poor medical documentation particularly with respect to basic information on dates, times and designation of the person making an entry in the casenotes.

- 15.1% of emergency assessment units included in the study did not provide access to 24 hour CT scanning. In 4.8% of the patients reviewed there was a delay in obtaining results of investigations which, in the view of the advisors, adversely affected the overall quality of care of some of them. For all patients, admitted as an emergency, there should be ready access to a full range of haematological and radiological investigations. The results of these should be rapidly available, and where necessary expert opinion should also be available, to assist the treating clinician in the interpretation of investigations.

- 68.8% of patients were under the care of consultants who had more than one duty when on call. These may have been consistent with their on call activity but even so 21.2% of consultants were undertaking more than three duties. On-take consultants, who have ultimate responsibility for emergency admissions, should make an initial patient review and subsequent reviews at time intervals which are appropriate for the severity of the patient's condition. These consultant reviews should be clearly documented in the casenotes.

- 12.4% of cases lacked documentary evidence of patients being reviewed by consultants following admission to hospital. Of further concern was that it was not possible, in nearly 50% of cases, to determine the time to the first consultant review due to lack of documentation. NCEPOD is of the view that in most cases the first consultant review should be within 12 hours from admission. Of the 496 patients where it was possible to determine the time to the first consultant review, 40% were not seen by a consultant within this time frame. Regular review by consultants is important because, due to working time constraints of trainee doctors, consultants may be the primary source of continuity of care. As a result the consultant must act as the team leader and ensure that formal systems are in place so that crucial information regarding their patients is communicated between changes in shifts of trainee doctors.

Furthermore due to the current working time constraints of trainee doctors, resulting in reduced patient contact, there is concern that they are less able to recognise the critically ill patients and act decisively. Many examples of this were seen throughout this study.

- 6.8% of patients did not receive adequate clinical observations, both in type and frequency. A clear physiological monitoring plan should be made for each patient commensurate with their clinical condition. This should detail what is to be monitored, the desirable parameters and the frequency of observations. It was difficult to find clear evidence in this study that emergency admissions received this.

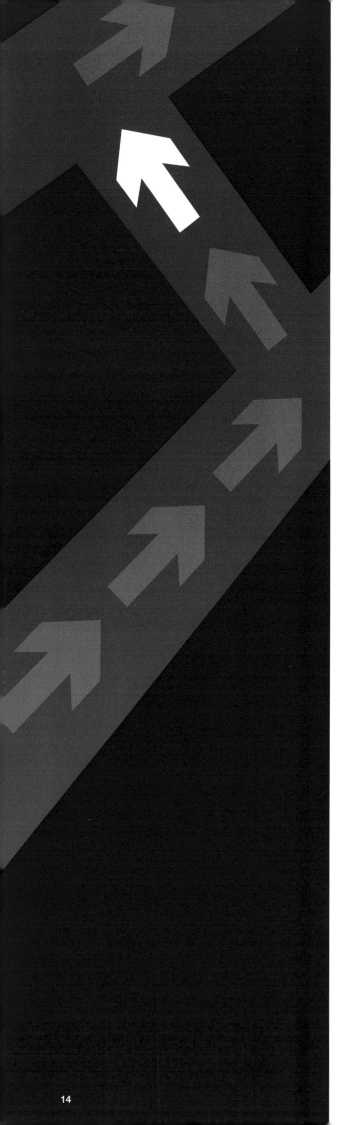

Principal recommendations

- The initial assessment of patients admitted as an emergency should include a doctor of sufficient experience and authority to implement a management plan. This should include triage of patients as well as formal clerking. The involvement of a more senior doctor should be clearly and recognisably documented within the notes.
(Clinical leads and heads of service)

- Patients admitted as an emergency should be seen by a consultant at the earliest opportunity. Ideally this should be within 12 hours and should not be longer than 24 hours. Compliance with this standard will inevitably vary with case complexity.
(Clinical directors)

- Documentation of the first consultant review should be clearly indicated in the casenotes and should be subject to local audit.
(Clinical directors)

- Trainees need to have adequate training and experience to recognise critically ill patients and make clinical decisions. This is an issue not only of medical education but also of ensuring an appropriate balance between a training and service role; exposing trainees to real acute clinical problems with appropriate mid-level and senior support for their decision making.
(Clinical directors)

- Consultants' job plans need to be arranged so that, when on-take, they are available to deal with emergency admissions without undue delay. Limiting the number of duties that consultants undertake when on-take should be a priority for acute trusts. *(Medical directors)*

- Hospitals which admit patients as an emergency must have access to both conventional radiology and CT scanning 24 hours a day, with immediate reporting. *(Medical directors and clinical directors)*

- Following the initial assessment and treatment of patients admitted as an emergency, subsequent inpatient transfer should be to a ward which is appropriate for their clinical condition; both in terms of required specialty and presenting complaint. *(Clinical directors)*

- Excessive transfers should be avoided as these may be detrimental to patient care. *(Clinical directors)*

- Robust systems need to be put in place for handover of patients between clinical teams with readily identifiable agreed protocol-based handover procedures. Clinicians should be made aware of these protocols and handover mechanisms. *(Heads of service)*

- A clear physiological monitoring plan should be made for each patient commensurate with their clinical condition. This should detail what is to be monitored, the desirable parameters and the frequency of observations. This should be regardless of the type of ward to which the patients are transferred. *(Clinical directors)*

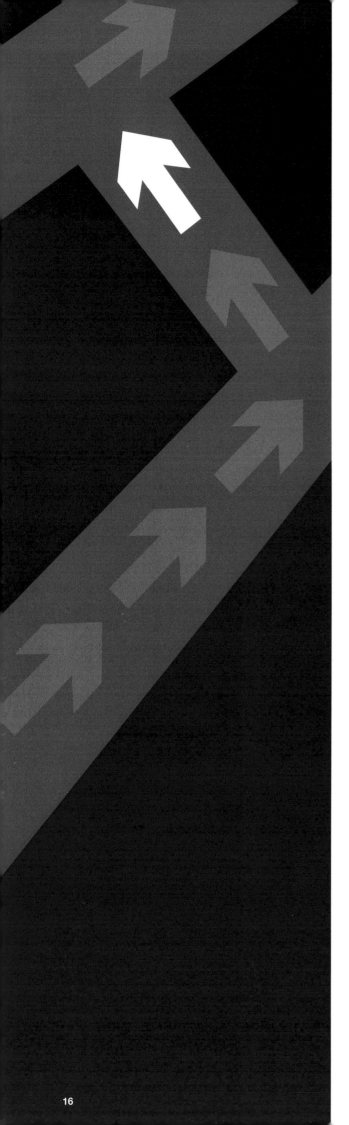

1. Method

Study aim

The aim of this study was to identify remediable factors in the organisation of care of adult patients who were admitted as emergencies.

Identification of indicators of care

No generic guidelines exist for the processes of care of medical and surgical emergencies. Consequently, a consensus group for this study defined a set of factors considered to be of potential importance in the organisation of care across the range of clinical specialties. This was carried out at a meeting held in May 2004 using consensus techniques.

1. Emergency admissions systems
   a) Appropriateness of location of initial assessment.
   b) Proportion of emergency admissions discharged home from the emergency department or Emergency Assessment Unit (EAU).

2. Access to investigations
   a) Availability of radiology and blood test results at the first consultant review.

3. Bed management
   a) Frequency of ward transfers.
   b) Appropriateness of first location post emergency department or EAU.

4. Time and timing of
   a) First review by consultant.
   b) Preventable adverse events.

5. Communication and information
   a) Access to pre-existing notes at first
      consultant review.
   b) Quality of handover between clinical teams.

6. Quality and quantity of staff
   a) Occurrence of daily medical assessment.
   b) Recording of appropriate observations.
   c) Consultant commitments whilst on-take.

Expert Group

A group of experts comprising physicians, surgeons, emergency department physicians, intensive care physicians, nurses, lay representatives and scientific advisors contributed to the design of the study and reviewed the combined analysis of the data, both from the questionnaires and the extra information from the advisor groups.

Study design

This study was conducted using both qualitative and quantitative methods of data collection from a selected group of patients. Peer review of each case was undertaken to identify possible remediable factors in the organisation of care using the indicators identified above.

Hospital participation

All relevant National Health Service hospitals in England, Wales and Northern Ireland were expected to participate, as well as relevant hospitals in the independent sector, public hospitals in the Isle of Man, Guernsey and the Defence Secondary Care Agency.

Within each site a named contact acted as a liaison between NCEPOD and the site, facilitating data collection and dissemination of questionnaires. This role is referred to as the NCEPOD Local Reporter.

Sample

An emergency admission is defined, according to the NHS Information Authority (NHSIA), as an admission that is unpredictable and at short notice because of clinical need, including via:

- **Emergency department or dental casualty department of the hospital;**

- **General practitioner: after a request for immediate admission has been made direct to a hospital, i.e. not through a bed bureau;**

- **Bed bureau;**

- **Consultant clinic, of this or another hospital (health care provider);**

- **The emergency department of another hospital where they had not been admitted.**

1. Method

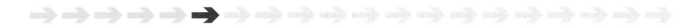

Sample selection

The Expert Group proposed a selection of patients that were thought most likely to test the processes of care during their hospital stay. All adult medical and surgical patients (≥16 years) who were admitted to hospital as an emergency admission on seven pre-determined days in February 2005 were considered and included if they met one of the following inclusion criteria:

- **Died on or before midnight on day 7 (following admission); or**

- **Were transferred to adult critical care on or before midnight on day 7; or**

- **Were discharged on or before midnight on day 7 and subsequently died in the community within 7 days of discharge.**

The selective nature of the sample must be borne in mind by the reader throughout this report, as this group was not representative of all emergency admissions.

Initially a sampling period of two days was allocated by NCEPOD and, to prevent bias, not publicised prior to data collection. The period was determined following an estimate of the total number of emergency admissions recorded by the Department of Heath's Hospital Episode Statistics, in order to produce a sample size of approximately 1000 cases. In fact this estimate proved to be inaccurate and led to an initial sample of only 342 usable cases. This was considered by the NCEPOD Steering Group to be inadequate and therefore the sampling period was increased to cover the whole week. A second wave of questionnaires was sent out to include those patients identified in the extended sample.

A list of all patients admitted as emergencies on the specified dates was produced by the NCEPOD Local Reporter. This list contained information on the admission and discharge codes, outcome at day 7 and the consultant whose care the patient was under, both on admission and on discharge.

For all included cases, questionnaires were sent to the relevant clinicians for completion. Additionally patients who were discharged on or before day 7 were identified for subsequent record linkage with the Office for National Statistics (ONS). NCEPOD supplied ONS with a list of those patients that had been discharged. ONS was then able to identify whether the patient was alive or had died within seven days of discharge. If the patient had died then the case was included as part of the study.

Exclusions

The following groups of patients were excluded from the study:

- **Patients who were brought in dead.**

- **Patients who died within an hour of arrival.**

This included mostly patients who arrived in a pre-morbid state for whom death was expected.

These groups were excluded because they did not allow any detailed analysis of the processes of ongoing care.

- **Patients whose prime reason for admission was for palliative care with a known terminal diagnosis prior to admission.**

This group of patients was excluded because of the complex intertwining of clinical and social care needs that brought about their admission to hospital.

- **Patients whose prime reason for admission was a psychiatric diagnosis.**
- **Obstetric cases (2nd and 3rd trimester).**

These patients were excluded because they fell into the remit of the other confidential enquiries. However, the study did include patients with an obstetric or psychiatric diagnosis where it was coincidental to the prime reason for admission e.g. a pregnant woman admitted with acute appendicitis.

Questionnaires and casenotes

The questionnaires were either sent to the NCEPOD Local Reporter to disseminate or directly to the clinician involved, depending upon the choice of the hospital. However, whichever method was used, NCEPOD requested that the completed questionnaires should be returned directly to NCEPOD.

There were three questionnaires.

1. Admission questionnaire

This questionnaire was sent to the admitting consultant. In this questionnaire NCEPOD requested information concerning the initial assessment, access to pre-existing medical notes, first consultant review, timely access to investigations, adverse events, ward transfers, handover between clinical teams, ward rounds and on-take commitments of consultants.

2. Ongoing care questionnaire

This questionnaire concerned information on appropriateness of first post-assessment location, ward transfers, adverse events, handover between clinical teams, ward rounds and on-take commitments of consultants. It was sent to:

- **The consultant under whose care the patient was on the day of death; or**
- **The consultant under whose care the patient was on day 7 at midnight, for those patients who went to critical care; or**
- **The consultant under whose care the patient was on the day of discharge (once death within 7 days had been established).**

If the patient was discharged or died before leaving the emergency department or the admission unit, only the admission questionnaire was required. Where the same consultant was responsible for the patient's management throughout the hospital episode both questionnaires were completed with specified sections of the ongoing care questionnaire excluded.

3. Organisational questionnaire

The organisational questionnaire was sent to the NCEPOD Local Reporter who facilitated its completion. This questionnaire concerned data on the assessment unit, numbers of patients admitted as emergencies and emergency admission protocols. For the purpose of this study 'organisations' were defined as a hospital or hospitals on the same geographical site. This allowed a better indication of the facilities available for a patient in the place where they were receiving care, rather than all the facilities available within a trust as a whole.

1. Method

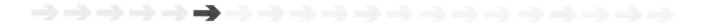

Copies of the following components of the casenotes were requested:

- **Admission notes. These included (where appropriate): initial clerking assessment, emergency department records, assessment unit records, last outpatient chart (if admitted from outpatients), and referral note from GP or other hospital;**

- **Casenotes from admission to day 7 (or less, where appropriate);**

- **Nursing notes from admission to day 7 (or less, where appropriate);**

- **TPR (Temperature, pulse, respiration) charts for day of admission to day 7 (or less, where appropriate);**

- **Investigations and blood test results;**

- **Drug charts.**

Advisor group

A multidisciplinary group of advisors was recruited to review the questionnaires and associated casenotes. The group of advisors comprised physicians, surgeons, emergency department physicians, intensive care physicians and nurses.

For each case reviewed, the advisor completed an assessment form (AF). This allowed both quantitative and qualitative analysis of the advisors' opinion. The AF was divided into sections based on the specific indicators of care.

Peer review process

All questionnaires and casenotes were anonymised by the research staff at NCEPOD. This included removing details relating to the patient, as well as the medical staff involved

and the hospital details. No clinical staff at NCEPOD or the advisors in a study had access to any information that would allow individuals to be identified.

Following anonymisation, each case was reviewed by one advisor within a multidisciplinary group. At regular intervals throughout the meeting the chair allowed a period of discussion for each advisor to summarise their cases and ask for opinions from other specialties or raise aspects of a case for discussion.

Data analysis

Following cleaning of the quantitative data, descriptive statistics were produced.

The qualitative data collected from the AF and free text answers in the clinical questionnaires were coded according to content and context. These data were reviewed by NCEPOD clinical staff to identify emerging recurring themes. Some of these themes have been highlighted throughout this report using case studies.

All data were analysed using Microsoft Access and Excel, within the NCEPOD offices, by the NCEPOD staff.

The findings of the report were reviewed by the expert group, advisors and the NCEPOD Steering Group prior to publication.

Quality and confidentiality

A number of pre-determined, mandatory key fields on each questionnaire had been set to ensure that data analysis could be performed effectively. If these key fields were not completed on receipt of the questionnaire by NCEPOD, the NCEPOD Local Reporter or clinician was contacted to see if these key data could be obtained.

Once the questionnaires were as complete as possible, the identifying casenote number on each questionnaire was removed.

The data from all questionnaires received was electronically scanned into a preset database. Prior to any analysis taking place, the dataset was cleaned to ensure that there were no duplicate records and that erroneous data had not been entered during scanning. Any fields that contained spurious data that could not be validated were removed e.g. double entries.

2. Overview of data collected

Hospital participation

One hundred and ninety two trusts or equivalent independent units contributed data to the study totalling 363 hospitals. Of the 363 hospitals that submitted patient data, 233 had patients that were eligible for the study. Additionally 201 organisational questionnaires were returned from sites that may or may not have had patients eligible for the study.

A total of 1609 admission and 1617 ongoing care questionnaires were returned to NCEPOD. Of these, 71 admission and 148 ongoing care questionnaires were excluded from the data analysis as they were either returned blank or were very poorly completed. Figure 2 illustrates the matches of questionnaires and/or advisor assessment forms (i.e. the denominator data) which were used for the data analysis.

Data returned

Figure 1. Overview of data returned

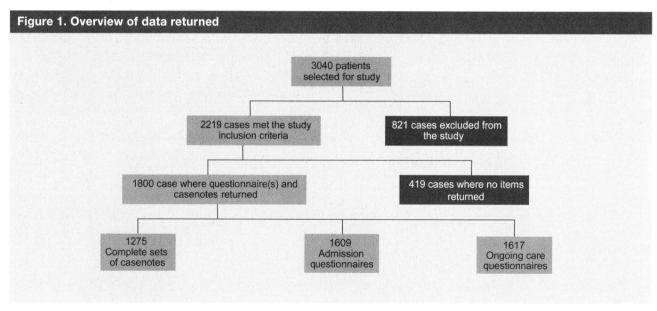

Figure 2. Denominators for analysis

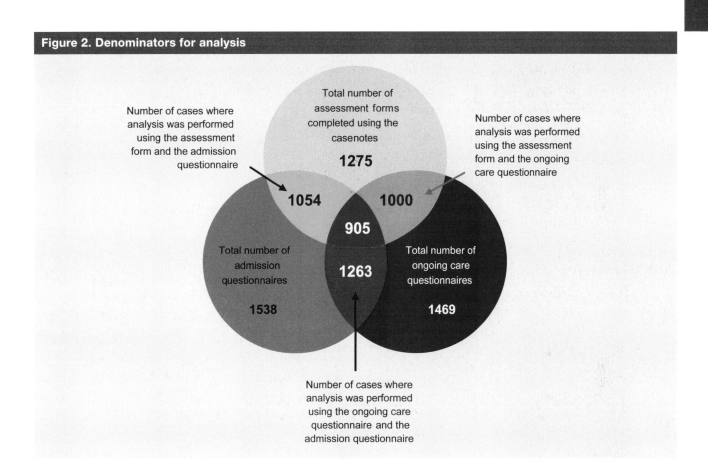

Number of cases where analysis was performed using the assessment form and the admission questionnaire

Total number of assessment forms completed using the casenotes

1275

Number of cases where analysis was performed using the assessment form and the ongoing care questionnaire

1054   **1000**

905

Total number of admission questionnaires

1263

Total number of ongoing care questionnaires

1538   **1469**

Number of cases where analysis was performed using the ongoing care questionnaire and the admission questionnaire

Age and gender

The patient sample was almost an even split of males (n = 638) and females (n = 634). In three further cases the gender of the patient was not recorded. The median age was 77 years and the females were slightly older than males (average age 74.5 versus 70.1 years).

Figure 3. Age range of patient sample

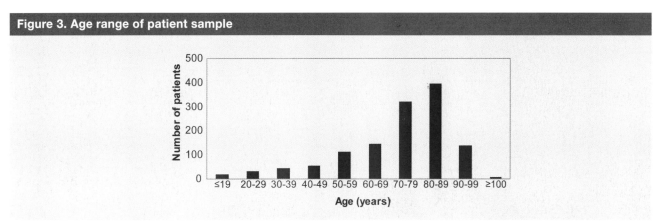

2. Overview of data collected

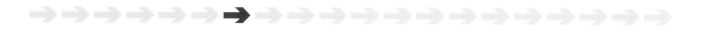

Route of admission

Approximately two thirds of patients were admitted after attending the emergency department and a further quarter of the sample were general practitioner (GP) referrals.

Table 1. Route of admission		
	Number of patients	**%**
Emergency department	817	66.2
GP	337	27.3
Emergency department at another hospital	53	4.3
Consultant clinic	23	1.9
Bed bureau	4	<1
Subtotal	**1234**	
Insufficient data	41	
Total	**1275**	

Medical and surgical admissions

More than three quarters of the patients in the study sample were medical patients.

Table 2. Type of admission		
	Number of patients	**%**
Medical	1186	78.5
Surgical	312	20.7
Medical/surgical	12	<1
Subtotal	**1510**	
Not answered	28	
Total	**1538**	

For the purposes of the data overview, day was taken to be from 08:00 to 17:59, evening from 18:00 to 23:59, and night from 00:00 to 07:59. Figure 4 shows the times of admissions within this categorisation. Unsurprisingly, the majority of admissions were during the day.

Time of admission

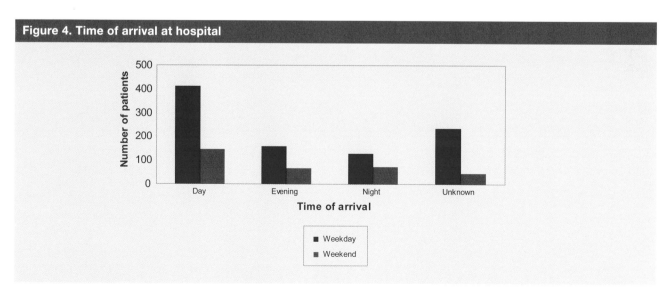

Figure 4. Time of arrival at hospital

Patient outcome

Approximately two thirds of the study sample (814/1275) died in hospital, and almost a third (415/1275) were admitted to critical care within 7 days of arrival. Of the three categories, relatively few patients died within 7 days of discharge from hospital.

Table 3. Patient outcome		
	Number of patients	**%**
Died in hospital	814	63.8
Critical care	415	32.5
Died in community	46	3.6
Total	**1275**	

Overall assessment of care

The advisors were asked to grade the overall care each patient received using the following categories:

Good practice: A standard that you would accept from yourself, your trainees and your institution.

Room for improvement: Aspects of **clinical care** that could have been better.

Room for improvement: Aspects of **organisational care** that could have been better.

Room for improvement: Aspects of both **clinical** and **organisational care** that could have been better.

Less than satisfactory: Several aspects of **clinical** and/or **organisational care** that were well below that you would accept from yourself, your trainees and your institution.

Insufficient information submitted to assess the quality of care.

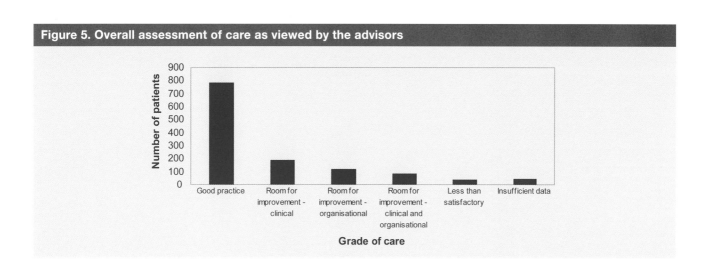

Figure 5. Overall assessment of care as viewed by the advisors

2. Overview of data collected

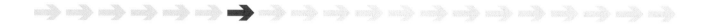

Figure 5 shows the overall quality of care of patients in the study as judged by the advisors. Encouragingly out of 1275 cases where the casenotes had been received 785 (61.6%) patients were believed to have received care consistent with good practice; in a further 405 (31.8%) patients the advisors considered that there were clinical/organisational areas for improvement and in only 39 patients was it believed that care was less than satisfactory.

It is important to note that for a large number of the patients in the sample (895/1469), upon admission, death was the expected outcome as noted by the clinician responsible for the patient's ongoing care. This is not necessarily inconsistent with good care. Thus, if a patient did not die in the 7 day period post admission this should not have positively influenced the advisors' overall assessment of the patient's care; as illustrated by Figure 6.

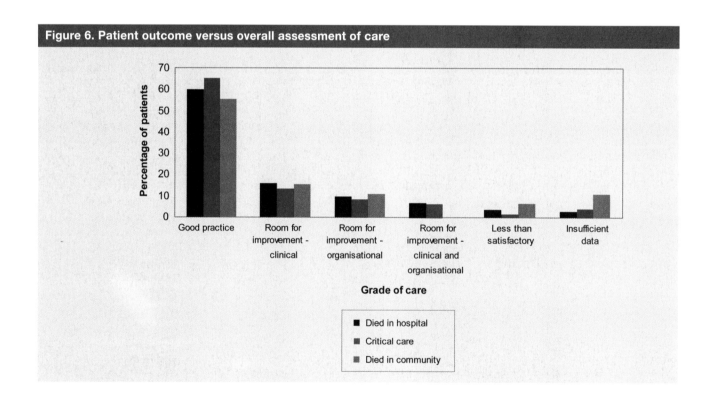

Figure 6. Patient outcome versus overall assessment of care

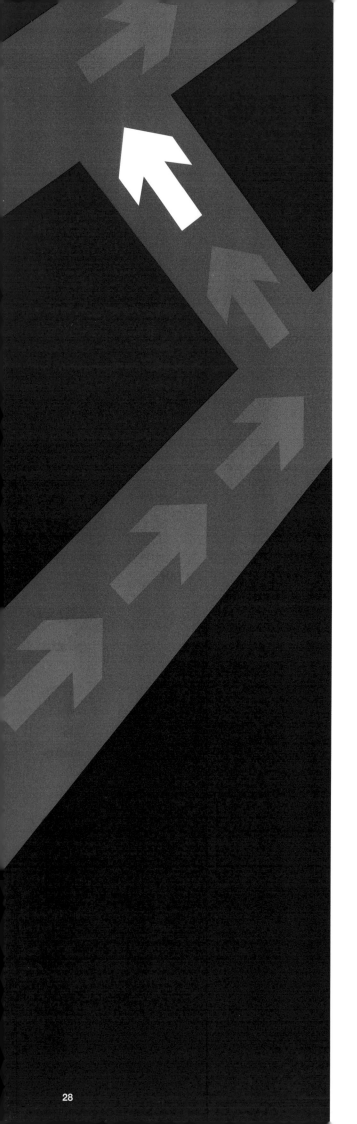

3. Results

This section presents and discusses the results of the study. Where remediable factors have been identified recommendations have been made.

Alongside the results, there is also discussion of the main issues that have emerged. References are made to guidelines where they exist and to the relevant literature. There are also illustrative case studies based on particular cases that highlight certain issues. Inevitably, many case studies illustrate what the advisors consider to be poor practice and indicate generic means of preventing such events in future.

3.1. Initial assessment

When a patient with an acute healthcare problem arrives in hospital he/she requires prompt clinical assessment, appropriate investigations and institution of a clear management plan. Furthermore, there should be early decision making to include involvement of relevant specialties and other required services followed by timely review by an appropriately trained senior clinician. This should be undertaken in an environment which best matches their clinical needs[8]. NCEPOD received organisational questionnaires from 201 participating hospitals to determine how this process was undertaken from both a clinical and organisational perspective.

Emergency assessment units

Although there is conflicting evidence on the optimal location for the assessment of emergency admissions, it has been recommended that these patients should undergo initial assessment in dedicated emergency assessment units (EAUs)[9,10].

An EAU has been defined as an area where adult emergency patients are assessed and initial management undertaken by inpatient hospital teams. The patient should only be in this area whilst early assessment is made and then moved either to another ward or discharged[11]. For the purposes of this study, the term 'EAU' is used as a generic term to include acute medical units, surgical assessments units and any dedicated emergency assessment unit outside of the emergency department or inpatient wards.

The rationale for the use of EAUs is that they can reduce both the emergency department workload and in-hospital length of stay. Patients can be seen sooner by a senior doctor, which will result in earlier decision making and so expedite treatment. This may improve patient outcome and satisfaction[12]. Standards set by the Society for Acute Medicine state that there should be a designated lead clinician and clinical manager in charge of an EAU[8].

The Society for Acute Medicine also recommends (personal communication) that every hospital which receives acute admissions should have an EAU which should be of sufficient size to accommodate, at least, the expected number of emergency admissions each day.

Furthermore, it has been recommended that acute trusts should ensure agreed clinical management policies for the assessment and initial care of emergency patients, and that these policies are known and observed[9].

Of the 201 hospitals from which an organisational questionnaire was returned, 23 did not have an EAU and a further five did not answer the question. The majority of the 23 that did not have an EAU were small specialist units or community hospitals that admit very few emergency patients. However, there were five large acute hospitals that indicated that they do not have an EAU. Of the remaining 173 hospitals, 96 had one EAU, 42 had two EAUs, 25 had three EAUs and 10 had four or more EAUs. The breakdown of the type of EAU is shown in Figure 7.

3.1. Initial assessment

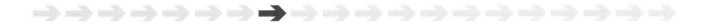

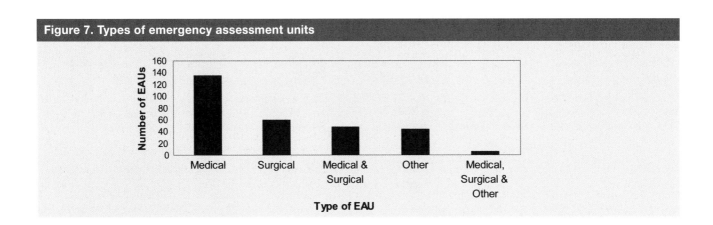

Figure 7. Types of emergency assessment units

Of those hospitals which had an EAU, 97.7% (169/173) had a medical and 60.1% (104/173) a surgical EAU. Examples of 'Other' as shown in Figure 7 included GP referral, trauma/orthopaedic and gynaecology. The relative proportions of specialty-specific EAUs would seem appropriate in view of the proportion of medical and surgical emergency admissions. An analysis of the location of EAUs revealed that 62% (185/298) of EAUs were separate from their emergency departments with 17% (51/298) being adjacent and only 8% (24/298) being part of the emergency department. It should be expected that sick patients will be able to access appropriate specialty care without prolonged transfer across hospital sites. Clearly, this may not be the case. While the data did not tell us exactly how far the EAUs were from their respective emergency departments, it does suggest that for the majority of patients there may have been some finite cross-site transfer.

NCEPOD found that in 5.7% (17/298) of EAUs there was no designated person in charge of the EAU. For these units to both run effectively in terms of good patient care and evolve and develop with respect to clinical standards someone should have overall clinical and administrative responsibility.

For hospitals that reported not having an EAU the inference must be that either these hospitals admit their patients directly to inpatient wards or undertake assessment in the environment of the emergency department where, owing to time constraints early discharge decisions may not be best facilitated.

For each EAU NCEPOD asked whether policies existed for patient clinical management, admission and discharge from the EAU. Out of the 298 EAUs 45 had no policies for patient management, 37 had no policies for admission of patients to the EAU and in 62 there were no policies for patient discharge from the EAU. Having clear policies in these important areas of patient care is essential to ensure EAUs function effectively and further work is required by trusts to meet the recommendations of the Royal College of Physicians of London's working party report[9].

Location of initial assessment

Using data from the admission questionnaire, NCEPOD identified that the majority of patients who were admitted as an emergency were initially assessed in the emergency department (972/1502) (Table 4). In 36 cases it was not recorded.

Table 4. Location of initial assessment

	Number of patients	%
Emergency department	972	64.7
Assessment unit	389	25.9
Outpatient clinic	18	1.2
Inpatient ward	98	6.5
Other	25	1.7
Subtotal	**1502**	
Unknown	14	
Not answered	22	
Total	**1538**	

This is consistent with, and reflects, the finding that 64.1% (817/1275) of patients were admitted via the emergency department. However, regardless of the location of the

initial assessment the overall quality of care, as graded by the advisors, was found to be similar.

NCEPOD identified that 6.5% (98/1502) of patients had their initial assessment on an inpatient ward. Additionally, of the hospitals that admitted these patients only one did not have an EAU. Thus the lack of EAU was not necessarily the reason why these patients were initially assessed on the ward. It is possible that they were admitted directly to an inpatient ward following GP referral and for certain specialties this may be appropriate (e.g. a prolonged epistaxis admitted directly to an ENT ward).

There was some variation in the location of initial assessment depending on the specialty of the consultant that the patient was admitted under (Table 5). There was a predominance of general medicine, care of the elderly, gastroenterology and respiratory medicine. In general, admission locations largely reflected the sub-specialty; for instance the majority of orthopaedic admissions 61/64 (95.3%) were via the emergency department.

Table 5. Location of initial assessment by most frequent consultant specialties

	Emergency department		EAU		Outpatient clinic		Inpatient ward		Other		Subtotal	Unknown	Total
		%		%		%		%		%			
General surgery	72	61	34	28.8	0		12	10.2	0		**118**	0	**118**
Orthopaedic surgery	61	95.3	0		0		2	3.1	1	1.6	**64**	1	**65**
Cardiology	61	63.5	16	16.7	6	6.3	12	12.5	1	1.0	**96**	2	**98**
Endocrinology	54	62.1	29	33.3	2	2.3	2	2.3	0		**87**	1	**88**
Gastroenterology	89	65.9	43	31.9	0		3	2.2	0		**135**	2	**137**
Geriatrics/ Care of the elderly	172	64.4	83	31.1	0		10	3.7	2	<1	**267**	0	**267**
Internal medicine	200	64.5	92	29.7	2	<1	12	3.9	4	1.3	**310**	6	**316**
Respiratory disease	77	58.8	47	35.9	1	<1	5	3.8	1	<1	**131**	3	**134**

3.1. Initial assessment

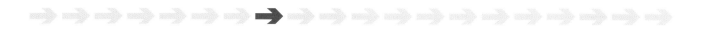

Quality of the initial assessment

The Royal College of Physicians of London recommends that a doctor with appropriate skills in acute medicine should be present at all times in all units receiving acute medical emergencies. This would usually be a specialist registrar, or equivalent, in medicine or in a medical specialty, who should have the MRCP(UK) Diploma or equivalent, and two years' recent experience in managing patients presenting as acute medical emergencies[13]. NCEPOD assessed the quality of the initial assessment and determined the designation of the healthcare professional making the assessment.

The advisors judged the majority of initial assessments to be good or adequate. However, in 90/1275 (7.1%) patients, the quality of the initial assessment was considered to be poor or unacceptable (Figure 8).

Of those patients where the initial assessment was considered poor or unacceptable, there was a greater proportion of patients where there was judged to be room for improvement in aspects of both clinical and organisational care, this is shown in Figure 9.

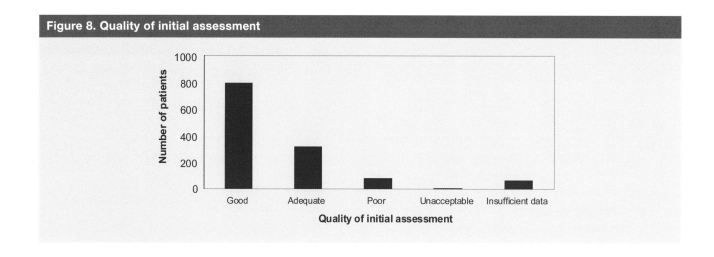

Figure 8. Quality of initial assessment

Figure 9. Overall quality of care of patients with poor or unacceptable initial assessments

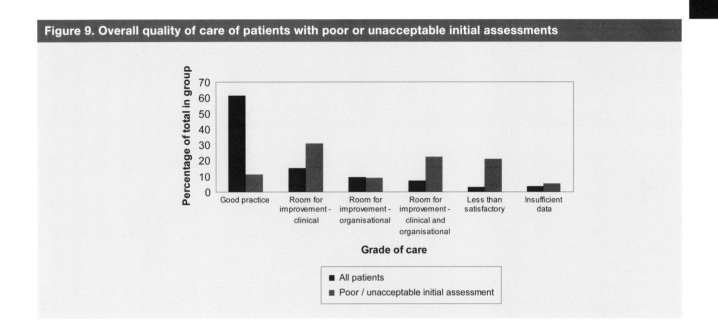

This finding suggests that the quality of the initial assessment may be associated with the overall quality of care of patients. While the data cannot be used to infer causality it is plausible that a poor initial assessment may lead to an incorrect or delayed diagnosis or engender delays in decision making and initiation of appropriate treatment.

NCEPOD found that the location of initial assessment did not influence the quality of the initial assessment as judged by the advisors (Figure 10). This would suggest that doctors provide an equal level of skill irrespective of the environment in which they make their clinical assessment.

The designation of the healthcare professional who undertook the initial assessment was determined from the admission questionnaire and casenotes and is shown in Table 6.

Table 6. Designation of initial assessor		
	Number of patients	**%**
Consultant	62	6.7
Staff grade	42	4.5
Associate specialist	5	<1
SpR 3	74	7.9
SpR 1/2	79	8.5
SHO	591	63.5
Nurse consultant	1	<1
Nurse practitioner	19	2.0
Other	58	6.2
Subtotal	**931**	
Unknown	29	
Not answered	94	
Total	**1054**	

3.1. Initial assessment

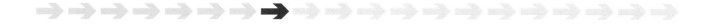

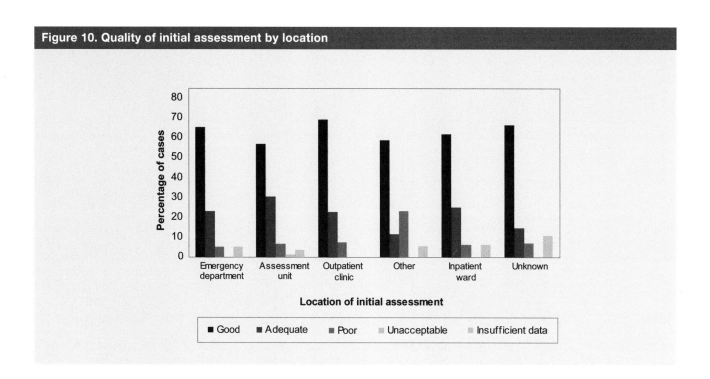

Figure 10. Quality of initial assessment by location

Where it could be assessed, these data show that 63.5% (591/931) of initial assessments were made by SHOs. This seemed to be at variance with that which has been recommended by the Royal College of Physicians of London[13] but may simply be a reflection of the selected sample. This notwithstanding, the proportion of poor or unacceptable assessments in this dataset was not different when the assessment was undertaken by an SHO as shown in Figure 11. It is likely that the question was interpreted as meaning the first clerking of the patient. First clerking by an SHO is regarded by the Royal College of Physicians of London as entirely appropriate, provided that timely more senior input is available, and that an appropriately senior doctor is involved in formulating the management plan.

It was often difficult to identify from the casenotes whether there was appropriate and timely senior involvement.

The quality of the initial assessment was no different between the different medical or surgical specialties. This indicates a uniform standard of practice and perhaps in turn reflects a uniformity of training.

Figure 11. Quality of initial assessment by grade of reviewer

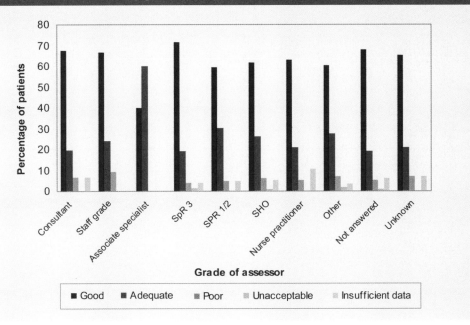

Quality of documentation

A recurring theme found by the advisors was the poor standard of documentation in the casenotes; the overall legibility of written entries being poor.

In many instances, entries were neither dated nor timed; nor was the designation of the person making an entry readily identifiable. For example, the initial clerking of a patient by an SHO may have been rapidly followed by senior input which was not recorded in the casenotes. Similar findings have previously been reported by NCEPOD, most recently in "An Acute Problem"[14] which identified that in 37% of casenotes reviewed the grade of the reviewer was not documented.

The advisors were also concerned that documentation of a management plan was incomplete or absent in a number of cases. This may make secondary decision making difficult

for doctors unfamiliar with the patient. It may also cause difficulty should there be a necessity for a retrospective justification of treatment e.g. in the Coroner's Court.

In contrast, the advisors were impressed and encouraged by the standard of nursing notes, which were generally better than the medical notes. The advisors also noted that there was an increasing number of proformae documents being used to aid record keeping. However, while these generally improved clarity there was a lack of standardisation which made identification of information more difficult. NCEPOD believes that caution is advisable in equating clarity of notes with better care. However, if proformae are to be used in healthcare records there is an argument that these should be standardised across the NHS. In accordance with this, NCEPOD has been made aware that the Royal College of Physicians of London[15] is developing a standardised clerking proforma to be used across all hospitals for the assessment of emergency medical admissions.

3.1. Initial assessment

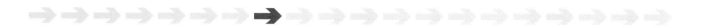

Case study 1 is one example of how a poor initial assessment can influence the final patient outcome.

Case study 1

A very elderly patient was admitted in the early hours of the morning to the emergency department with a fractured neck of femur following a fall at home. The patient had a past medical history of ischaemic heart disease and chronic obstructive pulmonary disease and was taking anti-failure medication. An orthopaedic SHO performed an initial assessment of the patient; with a cardiovascular and respiratory assessment being described as normal. Eight hours later the patient underwent a hemiarthroplasty performed by an orthopaedic SpR. None of the patient's cardiac medications had been given preoperatively because of a 'nil by mouth' order. There was no further entry in the patient notes from the initial assessment until a review in theatre recovery with postoperative shortness of breath and an arterial oxygen saturation of 75%. Postoperative treatment was given for cardiac failure and despite admission to intensive care and aggressive therapy the patient died two days later. A post-mortem was performed which showed that the patient had had an acute myocardial infarction which predated the admission.

The advisors judged the initial assessment to have been poor due to the brevity and lack of clarity of the clerking and minimal assessment of the patient's cardiac status. They commented that if more time and attention had been paid to the patient's clinical status in the preoperative period the acute myocardial event may have been identified and the patient's condition could have been optimised prior to surgery.

In contrast case study 2 highlights a good initial assessment.

Case study 2

An elderly patient was admitted with epigastric pain on a Friday morning via the emergency department to an EAU. The patient was seen by a surgical SHO who performed an initial clinical assessment and made a differential diagnosis of cholecystitis, peptic ulcer disease or small bowel obstruction. A clear plan of management was documented. The patient was reviewed by a consultant surgeon within six hours and an ultrasound was arranged the same day which showed a dilated common bile duct. A CT scan was organised for the next day. The patient's pain persisted with increasing abdominal distension. The CT scan showed small bowel obstruction. The patient was reviewed again by a consultant surgeon that day. The patient's general condition was judged to be deteriorating with increasing signs of sepsis. An emergency laparotomy was performed by the consultant surgeon. At operation a necrotic gall bladder was found with small bowel adhesions. A cholecystectomy and release of adhesions was undertaken. Postoperatively the patient was admitted to an adult ICU and required ventilatory and inotropic support due to persistent hypotension due to sepsis. However, within two days the patient was extubated and the sepsis had resolved. The patient returned to the ward two days later.

It was the advisors view that this patient received good overall quality of care and that the initial assessment was good and well documented. There was an appropriately timed first consultant review with continued daily consultant reviews. The patient had a timely operation and had good postoperative care on an adult ICU and despite the predictable complications, made a good recovery.

Key findings

- Of those hospitals that had an EAU 97.7% (169/173) had a medical EAU and 60.1% (104/173) a surgical EAU.

- The majority of initial assessments were made in the emergency department.

- The overall standard of initial assessment of emergency admissions was good or adequate but 7.1% (90/1275) were poor or unacceptable in the advisors' opinions.

- In 5.7% (17/298) of EAUs there was no designated lead clinician or clinical manager in charge of the EAU.

- In a significant number of EAUs there was a lack of policies related to clinical management, admission and discharge.

- The initial assessment of patients was frequently undertaken by SHOs.

- There were examples of poor medical documentation particularly in respect of basic information on the dates, times or designation of the person making an entry in the casenotes.

- The use of proformae in the casenotes aided the initial assessment but there was a lack of standardisation of the information recorded.

Recommendations

- Patients admitted to hospital as an emergency should be assessed in an area which has appropriate staff and facilities to allow early decision making and initiation of treatment. *(Clinical directors)*

- Emergency Admission Units should have a designated clinical and administrative lead and have policies for clinical management, admission and discharge of patients. *(Clinical directors)*

- The initial assessment of patients admitted as an emergency should include a doctor of sufficient experience and authority to implement a management plan. This should include triage of patients as well as formal clerking. The involvement of a more senior doctor should be clearly and recognisably documented within the notes. *(Clinical leads and heads of service)*

- The quality of medical note-keeping needs to improve. All entries in notes should be legible, contemporaneous and prompt. In addition, they should be legibly signed, dated and timed with a clear designation attached. *(Medical directors)*

3.2. First consultant review

There is general agreement that early senior clinician involvement in the management of patients admitted as an emergency can improve the quality of care. There is also evidence that more senior staff are less likely to make diagnostic errors, have a greater ability to recognise severely ill patients and are better able to make clinical management plans[16]. There has been concern raised by the National Patient Safety Agency[27] that trainees are less able to recognise severely ill or deteriorating patients and that this may have a detrimental effect on outcome. Concerns regarding the recognition of acutely ill patients have also been highlighted in recent guidelines by the National Institute for Health and Clinical Excellence[28]. Thus the timing of the first contact that a patient has with a consultant may have a major influence on the quality and standard of care the patient receives.

Using the casenotes, NCEPOD attempted to determine the time from a patient arriving in hospital to the time they were seen by a consultant.

NCEPOD could find no evidence of any consultant review in 12.4% (158/1275) of cases. In 53.5% (682/1275) of cases it was not possible to determine, from the casenotes, the time of the first consultant review and thus it was not possible to calculate the time from the patient's arrival into hospital to the time the patient was first reviewed by a consultant. However, in several of these cases the clinician completing the questionnaire indicated that the patient had been reviewed by a consultant. It is of considerable concern that this was not documented. It may be important for trainees making subsidiary management decisions to be able to recognise that specific consultant input has already been given and a senior level management plan instituted. This in turn, may help trainee doctors to make rational and appropriate decisions in difficult situations e.g. end of life decisions. Advisors commented that there was both a great deal of evidence that junior/trainee doctors were 'asked to see patient' without having had previous input and there was a general reluctance for juniors to make decisions and act.

There appears to have been an improvement on the findings of "An Acute Problem"[14] where only 9% of casenotes displayed evidence of patients being reviewed by a consultant. Although, a different sample of patients was investigated it is encouraging that more emphasis seems to have been given to recording this important component of patient care since the publication of this NCEPOD report.

Patients were more frequently first reviewed by a consultant following admission to an EAU compared with other locations as shown in Figure 12. This contrasts with the frequency of initial assessment of the patient occurring in the emergency department and would indicate that patients have moved through the initial admission process on to the next stage of clinical care.

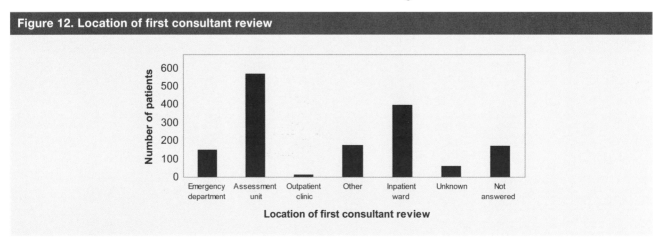

Figure 12. Location of first consultant review

Of the 496 cases where NCEPOD could determine the time to the first consultant review, 458 patients had their first consultant review within 24 hours (Figure 13) of admission, which is in keeping with the standard laid down by the Royal College of Physicians of London. Their recommendation is that 90% of patients should be reviewed by a consultant within 24 hours of admission[17].

However, in the intensive care setting it has been recommended that acutely ill patients should be seen by critical care consultants within 12 hours of admission[17]. Furthermore, it has also been suggested that senior doctors should review such patients within an hour of referral from the emergency department[18,19].

It was the view of the advisors that the majority of patients admitted as an emergency should be seen by a consultant within 12 hours where appropriate. Using this standard, 39.9% (198/496) of patients were not reviewed within this timeframe. However, this may not have been inappropriate as the necessity for early consultant review is entirely dependant on the nature and clinical severity of the patient's condition. For instance in medical EAUs, the 24 hour consultant review standard may be sufficient for the majority of patients. Whereas, there will be a subgroup, the critically ill, that will require early consultant review to ensure that a correct diagnosis has been made and that appropriate treatment has been initiated. Early review of these patients may allow appreciation of the severity of their clinical condition thus identifying the necessity for review and possible transfer to Level 2/3 care. Even then it may be arguable (with the exception of the rapidly deteriorating patient) that results should be available before a secondary management decision is made e.g. arterial blood gas results in a patient with severe pneumonia.

Figure 13. Time to first consultant review

8% of patients had not been seen at 24 hours

40% of patients had not been seen at 12 hours

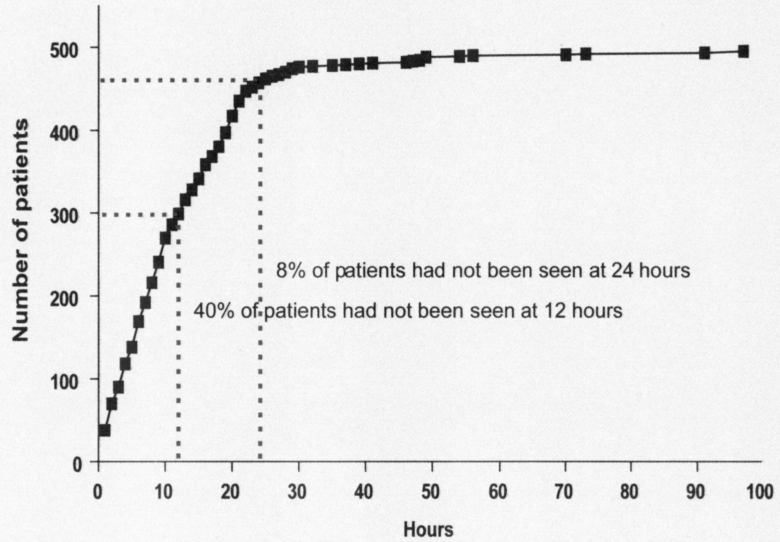

3.2. First consultant review

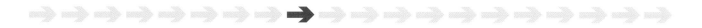

The advisors were asked, based on the clinical needs of the patient, whether the time to the first consultant review was acceptable, the answers are shown in Table 7.

Table 7. Was the time to first consultant review acceptable?		
	Number of patients	**%**
Yes	521	83.9
No	100	16.1
Subtotal	**621**	
Unable to assess	654	
Total	**1275**	

Of the 100 patients where the time to the first consultant review was judged to be unacceptable, the review was 12 hours or more from arrival in the hospital in 45 cases. However, these data should be considered with the knowledge that for nearly half 47.7% (609/1275) of the patients, the advisors were unable to form an opinion

on the acceptability of review as there was deemed to be insufficient information within the casenotes to identify the time the patient was seen.

Of the cases that could be assessed, there were 16.1% (100/621) of patients where the advisors judged that the time to the first consultant review was unacceptable.

Following on from this, the time of day, and the day of the week of admission of these 100 patients was also determined. No difference was detected in the time from arrival to first consultant review in relation to either time or day of arrival. It is encouraging that regardless of the time of admission the advisors did not judge that there was an excess of unacceptable delays.

Of those patients where the time to the first consultant review was deemed unacceptable, the overall quality of care was generally less good compared with the complete dataset as shown in Figure 14. However, caution should be used in drawing inferences, where comparisons between multiple advisors' views are being made.

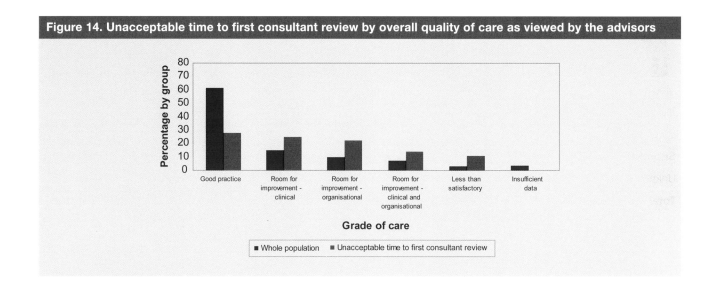

Figure 14. Unacceptable time to first consultant review by overall quality of care as viewed by the advisors

The reasons why the advisors considered these patients to have received less than good overall quality of care was further explored. Of the 100 patients where the time to the first consultant review was unacceptable, the advisors were asked if, in their opinion, this delay affected the diagnosis (Table 8) or outcome (Table 9).

The time to first consultant review was also compared with specialty. The specialty of the consultant could only be established for those cases in which an admission questionnaire, in addition to the casenotes, had been returned and is shown in Table 10. Of the 621 cases where the time to first consultant review could be assessed, 533 could have a specialty identified. There appeared to be a proportionally greater representation from the medical specialties compared with the surgical specialties.

Table 8. Did the unacceptable review time affect diagnosis?

	Number of patients	%
Yes	31	32.6
No	64	67.4
Subtotal	**95**	
Insufficient data	5	
Total	**100**	

Table 9. Did the unacceptable review time affect outcome?

	Number of patients	%
Yes	45	49.5
No	46	50.5
Subtotal	**91**	
Insufficient data	9	
Total	**100**	

Table 10. Medical and surgical specialty patients where the time to the first consultant review was unacceptable

	Time to consultant review acceptable?						
	Yes	%	No	%	Subtotal	Unable to assess	Total
Medical	367	87.2	54	12.8	**421**	414	**835**
Medical/Surgical	4	80	1	20	**5**	5	**10**
Surgical	81	75.7	26	24.3	**107**	86	**193**
Subtotal	**452**		**81**		**533**	**505**	**1038**
Unknown	6		2		**8**	8	**16**
Total	**458**		**83**		**541**	**513**	**1054**

3.2. First consultant review

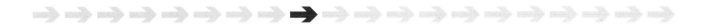

These data indicate that delays in the consultant reviewing patients following admission may have a detrimental effect on the patient outcome. Examples of effects on outcome include an admission to intensive care that could have been averted, an adverse alteration in prognosis, or an avoidable death.

The advisors were also asked if the consultant making the first review was of an appropriate specialty for the patient's condition. In 57/823 (6.9%) patients where the specialty was recorded, the advisors considered that the specialty of the consultant was inappropriate as shown in Table 11.

The overall quality of care for patients who were not seen by a consultant of an appropriate specialty appeared, in this dataset, to be marginally less good compared to the complete dataset. As mentioned above, the comparisons made here were between multiple advisors' views and any inferences must be viewed with caution. These data are presented in Figure 15.

Table 11. Was the consultant of an appropriate specialty?		
	Number of patients	**%**
Yes	766	93.1
No	57	6.9
Subtotal	**823**	
Unable to assess	452	
Total	**1275**	

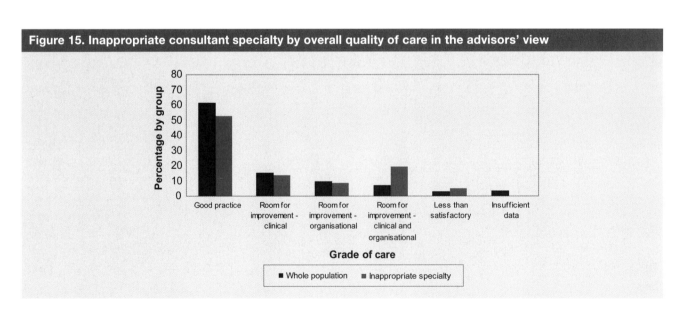

Figure 15. Inappropriate consultant specialty by overall quality of care in the advisors' view

The advisors were asked whether the fact that the patient was reviewed by a consultant of an inappropriate specialty had an effect on the patient's diagnosis (Table 12) or outcome (Table 13).

Table 12. Did the inappropriate specialty affect diagnosis?		
	Number of patients	**%**
Yes	13	23.6
No	42	76.4
Subtotal	**55**	
Insufficient data	2	
Total	**57**	

Table 13. Did the inappropriate specialty affect outcome?		
	Number of patients	**%**
Yes	16	32.7
No	33	67.3
Subtotal	**49**	
Insufficient data	8	
Total	**57**	

For approximately a quarter of these patients, the advisors considered that the diagnosis was affected and in a third the outcome was affected.

This would indicate that it is more important that patients be seen by a consultant within a reasonable timeframe determined by their clinical condition rather than by a consultant of appropriate specialty. This would support the view that delays in seeing a doctor of adequate seniority and experience may have a detrimental effect on patient care.

There were many examples in the cases reviewed by advisors of poor or absent decision making by trainees. Furthermore, there were instances of trainees underestimating the severity of patients' physiological dysfunction. Many of these patients had delays in their diagnosis, which, in the advisors' opinion, resulted in delayed definitive care and a worse outcome.

Good Surgical Practice[20] states that "it is the responsibility of surgeons to delegate assessment or emergency surgical operations only when they are sure of the competence of those trainees and non-consultant career grades to whom the patient's operative care will be delegated." Furthermore the Royal College of Physicians of London recommends that "an appropriately trained member of the clinical staff should assess according to clinical need, and certainly within four hours of arrival, all patients presenting to hospital as acute medical emergencies. This should include the development of a management plan. A consultant physician who has no other scheduled commitments should support this doctor and that 15 minutes for each new patient should be available on a consultant's 'post-take' ward round. This equates to about one clinical four hour programmed activity for a consultant to see sixteen new emergency admissions"[13].

NCEPOD is concerned that in the examples cited, these recommendations have not been followed.

Overleaf, case studies 3, 4 and 5 provide examples of cases that illustrate some of the issues highlighted in this section of the report.

3.2. First consultant review

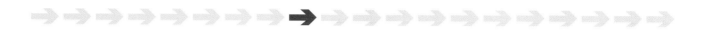

Case study 3

A young patient was admitted with right loin pain under the Urologists. Although not shocked on admission the patient gradually deteriorated displaying features consistent with insidious septic shock. Reviews were undertaken by several trainees but no review by an appropriate surgeon was made until 24 hours post-admission. The result of a previously performed CT scan was unavailable to the reviewing surgeon. The first consultant review was in theatre at laparotomy which revealed peritonitis secondary to a ruptured tubo-ovarian abscess. The patient was admitted to ICU postoperatively.

The advisors commented that this represented less than satisfactory care owing to a failure of trainees to act when the patient was clearly deteriorating.

Case study 4

A very elderly patient was admitted to the emergency department from a nursing home at 02:00 with pneumonia. The patient had a known history of ischaemic heart disease and Parkinson's disease. A medical SHO made a comprehensive initial assessment but no management plan was documented. The patient was not re-assessed again until the first consultant review 17 hours after arrival in the emergency department. By this time the patient had deteriorated and had a heart rate of 120 and a respiratory rate of 30 with overt signs of sepsis. Despite aggressive therapy with IV antibiotics the patient died 24 hours later.

The advisors were of the opinion that the lack of a clear management plan on admission, and the long duration to the first consultant review, delayed the initiation of medical treatment and contributed to the patient's eventual demise.

Case study 5

An elderly patient was admitted via the emergency department at 13:00 on a week day feeling unwell. Initial observations revealed a pulse of 140 beats per minute and blood pressure was 102/47mmHg. An ECG showed atrial fibrillation. A bedside glucose measurement at 14:00 was 33mmol/l. At 16:30 the patient was reviewed by a medical SHO, having been asked to see the patient because of the high glucose. The entry in the casenotes described the patient as a "newly diagnosed type I diabetic with diabetic ketoacidosis and secondary AF". The patient was started on a sliding scale of insulin, IV fluids and oral digoxin; then admitted to an acute medical ward. At 06:00 the next morning the nursing staff noticed, on turning the patient, that the patient's sacral area was inflamed. The patient had a persistent metabolic acidosis, pH 7.2 and pyrexia 39°C during the rest of that day. At 20:00 a medical SpR reviewed the patient and identified a "perianal abscess" and referred the patient to an anaesthetic SpR who diagnosed severe systemic sepsis. Following discussion with an anaesthetic consultant the patient was admitted to the ICU, intubated, ventilated and stabilised. A surgical opinion revealed an ischiorectal abscess. The patient underwent an urgent incision and drainage with radical debridement of fascia and skin. Unfortunately necrotizing fasciitis developed and the patient had repeated surgical debridements over the next few days. The patient was still on the ICU on day 7 of admission.

The advisors were of the view that the trainee medical staff failed to recognise the severity of this patient's condition and missed the infective cause for the diabetic ketoacidosis. If a more comprehensive initial assessment had been made, and more frequent medical review performed, this patient may not have developed necrotizing fasciitis.

Key findings

- 60.1% (298/496) of patients were seen by a consultant within 12 hours of admission; 92.3% (458/496) were seen within the first 24 hours.

- In 12.4% (158/1275) of cases there was a lack of documentary evidence of patients being reviewed by consultants following admission to hospital.

- It was not possible to determine the time to the first consultant review in 47.8% (609/1275) of cases due to lack of documentation of time or date in the casenotes.

- Where times could be determined, the time to the first consultant review was unacceptable in 16.1% (100/621) of cases and, in the advisors' view, this had a detrimental effect on diagnosis and outcome in many of these patients.

- Early review by a consultant following admission to hospital is more important than being reviewed by a consultant of a specific specialty.

Recommendations

- Patients admitted as an emergency should be seen by a consultant at the earliest opportunity. Ideally this should be within 12 hours and should not be longer than 24 hours. Compliance with this standard will inevitably vary with case complexity. *(Clinical directors)*

- Documentation of the first consultant review should be clearly indicated in the casenotes and should be subject to local audit. *(Clinical directors)*

- Trainees need to have adequate training and experience to recognise critically ill patients and make clinical decisions. This is an issue not only of medical education but also of ensuring an appropriate balance between a training and service role; exposing trainees to real acute clinical problems with appropriate mid-level and senior support for their decision making. *(Clinical directors)*

3.3. Consultant commitments while on-take

The Royal College of Surgeons of England and the Royal College of Physicians of London recommend that consultants when on-take should give priority to emergency admissions. This may require them to organise their non-emergency fixed commitments so that they are available to assess and review every patient admitted as an emergency under their care during the on-take and post-take periods[17, 19, 20].

Prompt assessment and continuing review of acutely ill patients by senior clinicians improves continuity of care and decision making and ensures adequate supervision of trainees[9].

NCEPOD asked consultants completing a questionnaire to indicate their additional duties when on-take. It should be noted that some consultants completed more than one questionnaire.

One third (427/1370) of patients were under the care of consultants whose sole responsibility was the care of emergency admissions when on-take, but the remainder were under the care of consultants that had additional duties with 21.2% (298/1370) of patients under the care of consultants undertaking more than three duties when on-take as shown in Table 14.

Table 14. Number of duties of consultants when on-take (answers may be multiple)		
	Number of cases	**%**
1	427	31.2
2	365	26.6
3	280	20.4
4	200	14.6
5	84	6.1
6	11	<1
7	3	<1
Subtotal	**1370**	
Not answered	168	
Total	**1538**	

It has been previously stated that consultant surgeons should accept responsibility for the assessment and continuing care of every emergency patient admitted under their name. They should be available either within the hospital or within a reasonable distance of the hospital to give advice throughout the duty period and ensure that they are able to respond promptly to a call to attend to an emergency patient[20]. Figure 16 shows the number of duties by the medical and surgical specialties caring for the patients in this study.

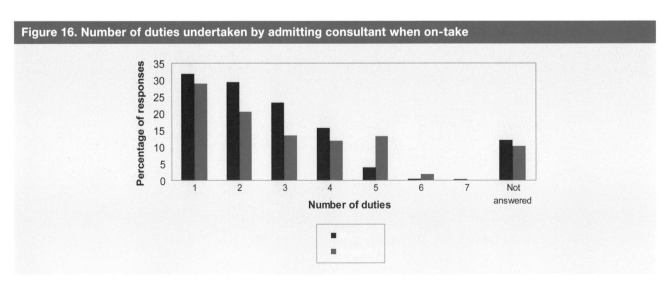

Figure 16. Number of duties undertaken by admitting consultant when on-take

Inspection of these data revealed that there was a high proportion of patients under medical consultants that had two to three additional duties while on-take and there was a high proportion of patients under surgical consultants who had five or more duties. While some of these duties may have been related to the management of emergency admissions, NCEPOD questions how a consultant with multiple duties when on-take can give adequate attention to the care of patients admitted as an emergency.

The types of additional duties undertaken are shown in Table 15. There may be instances where these additional duties do not necessarily impact on emergency care. For example, during their on-take period, a surgeon may undertake an elective operating list which has the capacity to incorporate emergency cases; or a consultant gastroenterologist may undertake an elective endoscopy list on which they can accommodate upper gastrointestinal haemorrhage patients. Some specialties manage a very small number of emergencies and/or their on-take admissions may rarely require immediate attendance so it is impractical to provide protected time for consultants in all specialties. Job plans must be based upon the specific requirements of each specialty. Furthermore, there may be examples where semi-elective activity supports emergency activity; for instance an orthopaedic trauma list where the theatre time is electively set but the patients operated on are determined by the previous day's take. However, NCEPOD would be concerned if the reason that such a large number of consultants are undertaking multiple duties, many of which

are elective in nature, reflects the priorities of hospitals to manage elective waiting lists or due to private practice commitments rather than emergency admissions.

Table 15. Types of duties undertaken by consultants when they are on-take (answers may be multiple)

	Number of cases
Care of emergency admissions	1245
Outpatient clinic	573
Elective operating list	136
Inpatient ward care	900
Elective diagnostic & intervention	281
Other	151
Not answered	168

In recent years there has been much discussion around the development of "acute physicians" to manage patients in the first 24 hours of hospital care. The Royal College of Physicians of London have set a target of three acute medical physicians in every acute hospital by 2008. The advent of Modernising Medical Careers has opened a specific career path for these consultants. NCEPOD would support this initiative but suggest there may be a similar need for an "acute surgeon" of consultant status. The precise role of the acute surgeon has yet to be defined but would include acute surgical evaluation and triage to appropriate surgical sub-specialties[13, 21-23].

3.3. Consultant commitments while on-take

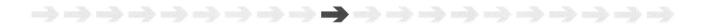

Key findings

- 68.8% (943/1370) of patients were under the care of consultants who had more than one duty when on call. These may be consistent with their on call activity but even so, 21.2% (298/1370) of consultants were undertaking more than three duties.

- Some consultants undertake non-emergency clinical care while on-take and this may have delayed their response to the management of emergency admissions.

Recommendation

- Consultants' job plans need to be arranged so that, when on-take, they are available to deal with emergency admissions without undue delay. Limiting the number of duties that consultants undertake when on-take should be a priority for acute trusts. *(Medical directors)*

3.4. Necessity for admission

Rapid and effective diagnosis ensures that some patients can be treated and discharged home rather than being transferred to an inpatient ward where further medical input may be superfluous. This is clearly an appropriate use both of the emergency admission unit (EAU) and hospital resources as well as medical time. It also has potential benefits for patients with respect to outpatient treatment and reduced exposure to hospital acquired infections.

Senior involvement, preferably at consultant level, facilitates this process by ensuring that an early decision is made as to whether the patient requires admission to an inpatient ward. This provides another example of early consultant involvement producing benefits for patient care. EAUs provide an appropriate environment to assess patients' requirements for admission or transfer.

Emergency admissions during February 2005

NCEPOD asked hospitals that admitted patients as an emergency for the total number of emergency admissions during the month of February 2005. A total of 214,249 patients were admitted as an emergency to 182 hospitals. From the 201 organisational questionnaires returned, 19 hospitals were unable to answer this question.

Of the 1275 patients included in this study and reviewed by advisors, 75 admissions (5.9%) were considered unnecessary. This is not a figure that can be easily ignored especially when one considers it within the context of the total number of emergency admissions per annum. Of the 75 unnecessary admissions there was no difference in their time of arrival or grade of initial reviewer compared to the necessary admissions.

A common theme amongst these unnecessary admissions was that of elderly patients admitted for social reasons or patients with untreatable terminal conditions which could have been adequately managed in the community.

Advisors were of the opinion that assuming appropriate community resources and support were available, many of these admissions might have been avoided, resulting in better patient care than provided in hospital.
A multidisciplinary approach involving palliative care teams and primary care services would facilitate community care.

3.4. Necessity for admission

Case study 6 gives an example of the type of admission that could have been avoided with appropriate resources.

Case study 6

A very elderly patient was admitted to the emergency department on a Friday evening from a nursing home after a fall. A history of complex medical problems including ischaemic heart disease, type II diabetes and bilateral varicose leg ulcers was noted. This initial assessment was made by a medical SHO who diagnosed chronic infected leg ulcers and prescribed oral antibiotics. There were frequent entries in the notes by the nursing staff over the next 48 hours stating that the patient was "comfortable". The next entry by the medical staff was at 08:00 on the following Monday at the first consultant review which stated that the patient was ready for discharge back to the nursing home.

The advisors commented that this admission was unnecessary. It was unclear why this patient presented to the emergency department on a Friday evening with a long standing medical problem that should have been managed in the community. One has to speculate that the admission was for social rather than medical reasons. It was the advisors' opinion that earlier senior medical involvement could have prevented this admission.

Key findings

- **5.9% (75/1275) of emergency admissions were considered unnecessary.**

- **Most of the unnecessary admissions were for patients who could have been cared for in the community.**

Recommendation

- **Appropriate mechanisms, both in terms of community medicine and palliative care, should be in place so that unnecessary admissions can be avoided.** *(Primary care trusts and strategic health authorities)*

3.5. Availability of investigations and notes

Availability of investigations in the first 24 hours

Access to modern basic investigations and the timely return of results are both essential to ensure rapid diagnosis and treatment in the acutely ill patient. Comprehensive investigation, coupled with patient monitoring and appropriate treatment services should be provided for all emergency patients[9]. In addition, it has been stated that assessment and treatment should not be delayed because of the absence of diagnostic or specialist advice[4]. This is relevant to all acute admissions but particularly to deteriorating patients where rapid investigations may be required to establish the diagnosis.

Additionally, one of the key causes of delayed discharge is the wait for the results of investigations[11].

NCEPOD enquired about 24 hour access by hospitals and emergency assessment units (EAUs) to conventional radiology, CT scanning, biochemical and haematological investigations with particular references to the availability of the results. These data were obtained from the admission and organisational questionnaires.

Access to investigations in the 173 respondent hospitals is shown in Table 16. Two of the respondent hospitals claimed not to have access to basic haematological and biochemical investigations. This calls in to question whether these units should be accepting acute admissions. In addition, NCEPOD discovered that 3.5% (6/173) of hospitals that answered the question did not have access to 24 hour conventional radiology and 21.1% (21/173) of hospitals that answered the question did not have access to 24 hour CT scanning.

Table 16. 24 hour access to investigations					
	Yes		No		Total
		(%)		(%)	
Conventional radiology	167	96.5	6	3.5	**173**
CT scanning	152	87.9	21	12.1	**173**
Haematology	171	98.8	2	1.2	**173**
Biochemistry	171	98.8	2	1.2	**173**

NCEPOD collected further data on the availability of investigations in individual EAUs. Access to investigations for patients admitted through the 298 EAUs is shown in Table 17 and Table 18. Again it is of notable concern that 7/298 (2.3%) of units did not have access to basic haematology and 9/298 (3%) to biochemistry. It is difficult to envisage how EAUs lacking access to these essential investigations can function effectively. Furthermore, the lack of access to 24 hour conventional radiology in 20/298 (6.7%) and 24 hour CT scanning 45/298 (15.1%) was of considerable concern to the advisors. It is regrettable that 21st century medicine in a developed country cannot provide such basic radiology and that cross-sectional imaging appears also to be at a premium; especially in the acute setting where accurate diagnostic techniques should be available to all clinicians.

3.5. Availability of investigations and notes

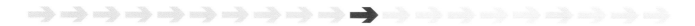

Table 17. Access to investigation in EAUs					
	Yes		No		Total
		(%)		(%)	
24 hour conventional radiology	278	93.3	20	6.7	**298**
CT scanning	253	84.9	45	15.1	**298**
Haematology	291	97.7	7	2.3	**298**
Biochemistry	289	97.0	9	3.0	**298**

Table 18. Access to radiological investigations by type of EAU		
Type of assessment unit	Units without 24 hour access to CT	Units without 24 hour access to conventional x-ray
Medical	21	7
Surgical	8	4
Medical & Surgical	2	1
Medical, Surgical & Other	1	0
Other	13	8
Total	**45**	**20**

NCEPOD also assessed whether the results of investigations ordered were returned in a timely fashion. The advisors were asked whether, in their opinion, there had been an unreasonable delay in obtaining results. They judged that there was a delay in obtaining the results of investigations requested in 4.8% (61/1275) of patients. Owing to poor documentation, it was not possible for the advisors to form an opinion in a further 15.1% (193/1275) of patients.

For the 61 patients for whom a delay had been identified, the advisors were further asked whether the delay had had a deleterious effect on the patients' diagnosis (Table 19) or outcome (Table 20). The advisors judged that in 32 (66.7%) cases the delay had adversely affected the diagnosis and in 27 (61.4%) cases it had adversely affected the outcome although this did not necessarily mean that these patients would have survived or not been referred to critical care had there not been a delay.

Table 19. Did the delay affect the diagnosis?		
	Number of patients	%
Yes	32	66.7
No	16	33.3
Subtotal	**48**	
Unable to assess	13	
Total	**61**	

Table 20. Did the delay affect outcome?		
	Number of patients	%
Yes	27	61.4
No	17	38.6
Subtotal	**44**	
Unable to assess	17	
Total	**61**	

The overall quality of care of those patients for whom it was judged that there had been a delay in obtaining results was compared to the quality of care of the whole dataset (Figure 17). Again it is important to note that multiple advisors' views are being compared. However, this analysis implies that where a delay had occurred there was an increased likelihood of the patient being judged to have received less than good overall clinical care and also room for improvement in both organisational and/ or clinical factors. This finding supports the impression that delays in obtaining the results of investigations can adversely affect patient care. It must be of concern that there is evidence of both restricted access to, and delay in obtaining the results of basic investigations especially when this had an impact on the quality of care.

Case study 7 provides an example of how delays in obtaining the results of investigations can have a deleterious effect on patient care.

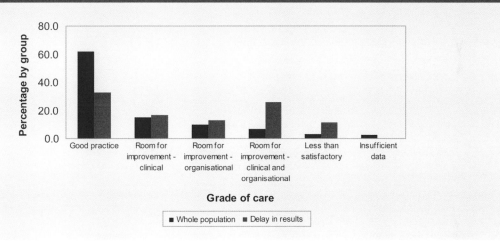

Figure 17. Delay in obtaining results by overall quality of care in the advisors' view

Case study 7

An elderly patient with known chronic obstructive pulmonary disease was admitted with an acute exacerbation secondary to a possible infective cause. The patient was considered to be "coping" by the pre-registration HO at the initial assessment. A chest x-ray was requested and oral antibiotics were commenced. Three hours after admission an arterial blood gas measurement revealed a pH 7.38, $PaCO_2$ 8.5 kPa and $PaCO_2$ 10 kPa on 28% oxygen. The chest x-ray was not performed until 12 hours after admission and the result not recorded in the notes until 24 hours post-admission. This showed left lower lobe collapse/consolidation and intravenous antibiotics were commenced. By this time

the patient's condition had deteriorated further and a review was conducted by an ICU outreach team which commenced non-invasive ventilation on the ward. Twelve hours later the patient was transferred to the ICU for close observation and still required non invasive ventilation on day 7 following admission.

The advisors considered the delay in obtaining and reporting on the chest x-ray was unacceptable. This delayed the decision to start intravenous antibiotics. Furthermore, if the results had been available more quickly it is possible that non invasive ventilation may have been instituted earlier altering the course of this ICU admission.

3.5. Availability of investigations and notes

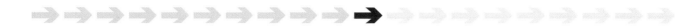

While it is important that investigations and results are readily available it is also important that clinicians use these resources wisely by not ordering inappropriate investigations. NCEPOD asked the advisors' opinion as to the appropriateness of the investigations undertaken. Reassuringly it was judged that in 92.5% (1127/1218) of patients all appropriate investigations were ordered. However, in 7.5% (91/1218) it was judged that some appropriate investigations had not been requested. Where there was thought to be an omission of appropriate investigations the advisors believed that it affected the diagnosis (Table 22) in 65/87 cases and the outcome (Table 23) in 48/77.

Table 21. Were appropriate investigations performed?

	Number of patients	%
Yes	1127	92.5
No	91	7.5
Subtotal	**1218**	
Insufficient data	57	
Total	**1275**	

Table 22. Did the omission of appropriate investigations affect diagnosis?

	Number of patients	%
Yes	65	74.7
No	22	25.3
Subtotal	**87**	
Insufficient data	4	
Total	**91**	

Table 23. Did the omission of appropriate investigations affect outcome?

	Number of patients	%
Yes	48	62.3
No	29	37.7
Subtotal	**77**	
Insufficient data	14	
Total	**91**	

Furthermore, when the overall quality of care of those patients who had not received all appropriate investigations was compared with the quality of care for the whole study sample it is possible that omission of investigations had a tangible detrimental effect (Figure 18). This is unsurprising, as it is to be expected that when relevant investigations are omitted then the quality of care a patient receives will be reduced.

In addition the advisors were asked whether inappropriate investigations had been ordered. In 94/1275 (7.4%) it was considered they had been.

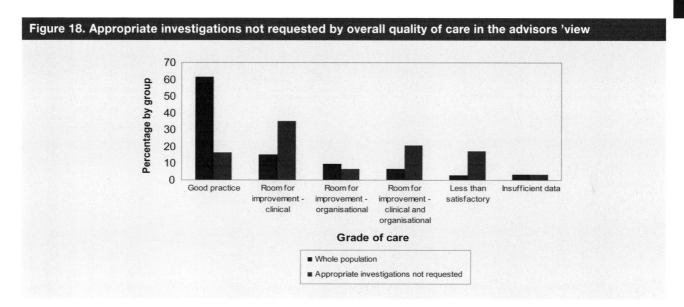

Figure 18. Appropriate investigations not requested by overall quality of care in the advisors 'view

These data lend some support to the assumption that omitting appropriate investigations has a deleterious effect on patient care. Unsurprisingly, there seemed to be no evidence that undertaking inappropriate investigations had a similar deleterious effect (Figure 19). In other words, over

investigation did not seem to cause harm. Nevertheless, one must surely argue that in a resource limited organisation such as the NHS, investigation requests should always have a clear rationale to justify them.

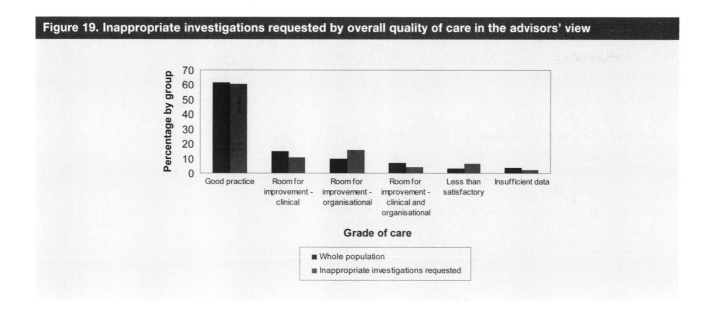

Figure 19. Inappropriate investigations requested by overall quality of care in the advisors' view

3.5. Availability of investigations and notes

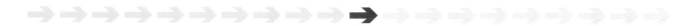

Examples identified by the advisors of inappropriate investigations included:

- **Chest x-ray in patient with no chest problems but terminal metastatic bone cancer;**

- **'Pointless' liver function tests in a terminally ill patient with a known diagnosis;**

- **Request for serum amylase in a patient with melaena.**

The advisors also commented on the poor recording of time and date of investigation results in the casenotes. This made it very difficult to be sure if real delays actually occurred, as the results may have been available to clinicians via other systems e.g. computers. However, it is important that the results and timings of investigations are clearly documented in the patient casenotes as soon as they are available. If this does not occur, vital information affecting patient care may be miscommunicated or lost.

Availability of casenotes

In only 12 instances did clinicians report delays in obtaining pre-existing notes. Examples of causes for these delays included:

- **Patient being treated at a different hospital.**

- **Trust kept notes off site because of storage difficulties.**

- **Old notes not available out of hours.**

Key findings

- Obtaining pre-existing notes did not seem to be a problem in this group of patients. This may be due to improvements in access to notes via medical records departments, or due to the fact that the pre-existing notes were not considered necessary.

- 15.1% (45/298) of EAUs that admitted patients as an emergency did not have access to CT scans 24 hours a day.

- 6.7% (20/298) of EAUs that admitted patients as an emergency did not have access to conventional radiology 24 hours a day.

- In 4.8% (61/1275) of cases there was a delay in obtaining results of investigations, adversely affecting the overall quality of care of some of these patients.

- In 7.5% (91/1218) of cases appropriate investigations were not performed.

- In 7.4% (94/1275) of cases inappropriate investigations were performed.

Recommendations

- Hospitals which admit patients as an emergency must have access to both conventional radiology and CT scanning 24 hours a day, with immediate reporting. *(Medical directors and clinical directors)*

- There should be no systems delay in returning the results of investigations. *(Clinical directors)*

- There should be a clear rationale for the ordering of investigations. Omission of appropriate investigations can have a deleterious effect on patient care. *(Lead clinicians)*

- All investigation results should be recorded with a date and time in the patient notes. *(Clinical audit)*

3.6. Transfers

During a hospital admission it is likely that most patients will be transferred between wards at least once. This is mainly a direct result of the advent of assessment units; patients being transferred from an area where they undergo initial assessment to a longer stay inpatient ward. It is then, perhaps, axiomatic that the ward a patient is transferred to should be one that can provide an appropriate environment of care for their condition. Using data derived from the admission and ongoing care questionnaires, advisor forms and casenotes, the appropriateness of the first inpatient ward that each patient was sent to, has been considered.

Doctors involved in the patients' ongoing care stated that 92.9% (1346/1449) of patients were admitted under an appropriate clinical specialty as shown in Table 24.

Table 24. Admission under an appropriate specialty

	Number of patients	%
Yes	1346	92.9
No	87	6.0
Unknown	16	1.1
Subtotal	**1449**	
Not answered	20	
Total	**1469**	

In addition, doctors responsible for the patients' ongoing care believed that 91.5% (1308/1430) of patients were transferred to an appropriate first inpatient ward with respect to their presenting condition as shown in Table 25.

Table 25. Was the first inpatient ward appropriate?

	Number of patients	(%)
Yes	1308	91.5
No	99	6.9
Unknown	23	1.6
Subtotal	**1430**	
Not answered	39	
Total	**1469**	

In comparison, only 6.9% (99/1430) of the patients in the study group were, in the opinion of the clinicians completing the questionnaires, sent to an inappropriate first inpatient ward for their condition.

When the same question was asked of the advisors, the figure for patients transferred to an appropriate first inpatient ward for their condition was deemed to be similar at 1059/1275 (83.1%) with 93/1275 (7.3%) thought to have been transferred inappropriately.

It is important that patients are not only admitted onto the correct inpatient ward but are also cared for by a consultant of the appropriate specialty. Data from this study shows that 95.9% (1255/1308) of patients admitted to an appropriate first inpatient ward were cared for by a consultant of a specialty appropriate for their condition. Reassuringly, in the opinion of the advisors, only 2.6% (38/1469) of patients were both admitted to an inappropriate inpatient ward and put under a consultant of an inappropriate specialty.

In the opinion of the advisors, 31/93 cases where the patient was admitted to an inappropriate inpatient ward were thought to have received care consistent with good clinical practice. However, 37/93 of these patients were thought to have received care that could have been improved by better organisation. This is an unsurprising finding as it is self-evident that better organisational control would place all patients on an appropriate ward. In 12/93 cases inappropriately placed patients were thought to have received less than satisfactory care. Despite this finding, it is perhaps heartening that a high proportion of patients were thought to have received good clinical care despite being placed on an inappropriate ward as shown in Figure 20.

Figure 20. Inappropriate first inpatient ward and overall quality of care in the advisors' view

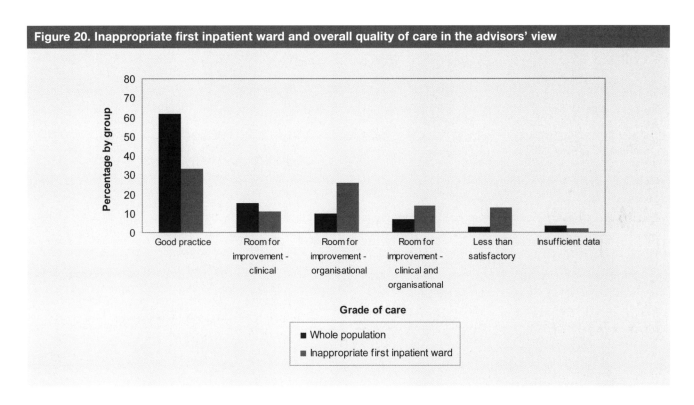

3.6. Transfers

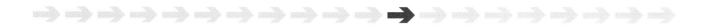

Case study 8 demonstrates an example of the effect on patients being admitted under an inappropriate specialty which can cause delays in diagnosis and treatment.

Case study 8

An elderly patient was admitted on a weekday afternoon to the emergency department with abdominal distension, pain and tenderness. The patient had been vomiting "brown sludge" for two days. An initial assessment by a medical pre-registration HO was carried out. In the clerking it was stated that the general impression of the patient was "fit and well" and the differential diagnosis was ascites possibly secondary to carcinoma. An abdominal x-ray was performed. In the early hours of the next morning the patient was reviewed by a medical SHO because of further vomiting and abdominal pain. The patient was noted to have an arterial oxygen saturation of 90%. A drink was allowed and a plan was made for an upper GI endoscopy. One day later a review was conducted by a medical SpR who reported the admitting abdominal x-ray as showing a sigmoid volvulus and referred the patient to the general surgeons. Thus the patient's first consultant review was at 48 hours post-admission by the surgeon. A diagnosis was made of large bowel obstruction and possible perforation. Intravenous fluid resuscitation was commenced and an urgent CT scan was requested. The CT scan confirmed the consultant surgeon's assessment and also showed liver and lung metastasis. The patient was taken to the operating theatre for a laparotomy. The patient's condition rapidly deteriorated in the immediate postoperative period. In view of his widespread metastatic disease it was decided not to undertake any further active management. The patient died four hours later.

Advisors were concerned that not only was there a delay in the patient being seen by a consultant but the medical trainees failed to recognise the severity of the patient's clinical condition. Why was this patient admitted under a medical service?
The failure to make a correct diagnosis, and to review and interpret the abdominal x-ray, resulted in an unacceptable delay in the patient being referred for surgical care. While the advisors accepted that this patient ultimately had a terminal condition, unnecessary discomfort may have been spared if appropriate action had been taken earlier.

It is a feature of modern emergency medicine that patients are likely to be transferred at least once during their admission. Often this is from the emergency department or emergency admission unit (EAU) to a ward. The number of transfers may also reflect protracted care pathways that might include, for instance, transfer from emergency department through EAU, theatre, intensive care and finally to a ward. NCEPOD found that 98.8% (1295/1311) of patients were transferred between 0 – 3 times; however 1.2% (16/1311) of patients were transferred between 4 – 8 times (Table 26). In the opinion of the advisors, 3% (38/1275) of transfers were considered excessive when all the prevailing circumstances were considered. Within this group of excessive transfers the advisors felt that in nine cases the diagnosis was affected by the excessive number of transfers. Furthermore they believed that in 18 cases the excessive transfers affected the outcome. While the absolute numbers are small it is of concern that such organisational deficiencies should be to the detriment of patients.

Table 26. Number of ward transfers		
	Number of cases	**%**
0	427	32.6
1	585	44.6
2	229	17.5
3	54	4.1
4	7	<1
5	5	<1
6	3	<1
8	1	<1
Subtotal	**1311**	
Not answered	158	
Total	**1469**	

Key findings

- The vast majority of emergency admissions in this study were sent to an appropriate inpatient ward.

- The vast majority of patients were looked after by a consultant of an appropriate specialty.

- However 12.9% (12/93) of patients placed on an inappropriate ward were thought to have received less than satisfactory care.

- Excessive transfers were thought to affect diagnosis and outcome in a small cohort of patients.

Recommendations

- Following the initial assessment and treatment of patients admitted as an emergency, subsequent inpatient transfer should be to a ward which is appropriate for their clinical condition; both in terms of required specialty and presenting complaint. *(Clinical directors)*

- Excessive transfers should be avoided as these may be detrimental to patient care. *(Clinical directors)*

3.7. Handovers

Handover of patient care is increasingly being recognised as central to safe patient management. It has been a core issue of the NHS Modernisation Agency's 'Hospital at Night' initiative. Using data obtained from the organisational questionnaire NCEPOD found that only 35.8% (72/201) of participating hospitals had an agreed protocol for handover, while 50.7% (102/201) did not. A further 7.5% (15/201) did not know whether such a protocol existed. Moreover, only 86% (733/852) of respondents who worked in a hospital with a written handover protocol were aware of the agreed handover procedure. This is revealing and suggests a serious deficiency both in the presence and awareness of these important protocols. As the study period was over two years prior to publication, it may be that protocols have been developed across the sites in the interim. Reassuringly, 86% (555/649) of respondents who worked in a hospital with no written handover protocol did have an agreed handover procedure. This is laudable and suggests that a responsible approach to handover is the prevailing attitude.

This study also investigated the handover of care between teams both following initial admission (in the emergency department or EAU) and subsequent to that once the patient had reached an inpatient ward. Data were obtained from the admission and/or ongoing care questionnaires. It was found that in 92.8% (1322/1425) of the admitted patients there was an agreed handover procedure between clinical teams (Table 27). The respondents were also asked whether there were any identifiable problems with team handovers during the initial admission. In only 1.3% (20/1538) of the admitted patients were such problems identified during the handover. In 4% (61/1538) of cases it was unknown if an admissions handover procedure existed.

NCEPOD also reviewed whether there was an agreed handover procedure between clinical teams subsequent to transfer to the first inpatient ward. It was found that in 93.6% (1262/1348) of cases in the study there was an agreed procedure for handover as shown in Table 28.

Table 27. Was there an agreed procedure for handing over care?

	Number of patients	%
Yes	1322	92.8
No	103	7.2
Subtotal	**1425**	
Unknown	61	
Not answered	52	
Total	**1538**	

Table 28. Was there an agreed procedure for handing over in subsequent teams?

	Number of patients	%
Yes	1262	93.6
No	86	6.4
Subtotal	**1348**	
Unknown	70	
Not answered	51	
Total	**1469**	

Respondents identified 1.4% (21/1469) of problematic handovers in this timeframe. This is clearly comparable with handover problems identified during initial admission. For approximately 4.8% (70/1469) of admissions, it was unknown whether there was an agreed handover procedure.

Generally, and reassuringly, handover problems seem to be small although it is perhaps surprising that agreed handover procedures are not more prevalent or identifiable in both groups; especially subsequent to initial assessment.

Key findings

- **50.7% (102/201) of hospitals did not have a written handover protocol.**

- **A proportion of clinicians were unaware of existing handover protocols.**

- **92.8% (1322/1425) of emergency admissions had a clear and recognisable handover procedure between clinical shifts both during initial assessment and subsequent to this.**

- **Handover-related problems appeared to be infrequent.**

Recommendation

- **Robust systems need to be put in place for handover of patients between clinical teams with readily identifiable agreed protocol-based handover procedures. Clinicians should be made aware of these protocols and handover mechanisms.** (Heads of service)

3.8. Reviews and observations

Clinical reviews

Good clinical care can only be provided following appropriate clinical review[17]. Advisors were asked to comment on the number of clinical reviews each patient underwent.

Where it could be assessed, in the advisors' opinion 93.2% (1122/1204) of patients had received adequate clinical review for their condition (Table 29). Of the 82 patients deemed to have been inadequately reviewed it was the advisors' opinion that in 27 cases this had adversely affected the diagnosis (Table 30), and in 50 cases the outcome (Table 31).

Table 29. Was the frequency of reviews appropriate?

	Number of patients	%
Yes	1122	93.2
No	82	6.8
Subtotal	**1204**	
Insufficient data	71	
Total	**1275**	

Table 30. If the frequency of review was not appropriate, did it affect the diagnosis?

	Number of patients	%
Yes	27	35.5
No	49	64.5
Subtotal	**76**	
Insufficient data	6	
Total	**82**	

Table 31. If the frequency of review was not appropriate, did it affect the outcome?

	Number of patients	%
Yes	50	72.5
No	19	27.5
Subtotal	**69**	
Insufficient data	13	
Total	**82**	

While the absolute numbers are small, they give an indication of the importance of appropriate clinical review in achieving a correct diagnosis and avoiding an adverse outcome. Furthermore, if a degree of conjecture were permitted, then the extrapolation of these figures over a one year period would perhaps suggest a more pressing issue.

When the appropriateness of reviews was assessed against the appropriateness of the specialty of the first inpatient ward it was found that if a patient was on an appropriate ward they received an appropriate review 88.8% (940/1059) of the time compared with 81.7% (76/93) if they were on an inappropriate ward. Reassurance can be gained from the insight that inappropriate placement does not necessarily mean patients are ignored. However, patient care should not be left a hostage to fortune and patients should be placed appropriately whenever possible.

Case study 9 is one example that illustrates how inadequate senior involvement and review can affect the quality of patient care.

Case study 9

A young patient sustained a head injury following a fall. On arrival in the emergency department a Glasgow Coma Score (GCS) of 10 was recorded and the patient was reported to be unco-operative. The patient was still in the emergency department 6 hours later when the patient fell off the trolley and hit their head during the fall. A CT scan was performed 11 hours after arrival in the emergency department which showed a left temporal contusion with a small amount of subarachnoid blood and minor midline shift. The patient was intubated, ventilated and sedated and transferred to the neurointensive care unit. First review by a consultant neurosurgeon occurred 20 hours after admission. An intracranial pressure (ICP) monitor was inserted. The patient was ventilated for three days and was seen once by a consultant neurosurgeon during this time. There was no repeat CT scan or cervical radiological investigation until day 4 of admission. The patient had a residual right partial hemiparesis on day 6 of admission.

The advisors were of the view that the trainee medical staff provided good care in stabilising the patient but were concerned that there was inadequate senior review and decision making.

Observations

The measurement of clinical observations, in an accurate and timely fashion, is central to all inpatient care. It is impossible to accurately assess a patient's health status unless there is regular recording of appropriate observations. Using the advisor assessment forms and clinical casenotes where supplied, the type, frequency and appropriateness of clinical observations were studied with respect to the patient's clinical condition and with respect to the patient's first inpatient ward.

In the cases where it could be assessed, the advisors were able to find clear evidence that 91.6% (885/966) of patients had received appropriate clinical observations for their condition. Additionally, in 23.5% (299/1275) of patients there was insufficient data to make a judgement. This illustrates that while patients may have been monitored correctly, it can often be difficult to assess this in retrospect which may have distinct medico-legal ramifications. It should always be clear from casenotes what observations have been undertaken. Moreover, the advisors recorded that 8.4% (81/966) of patients were found to have had inappropriate observations for their clinical condition which can be seen in Table 32.

Table 32. Were the clinical observations appropriate?

	Number of patients	%
Yes	885	91.6
No	81	8.4
Subtotal	**966**	
Insufficient data	309	
Total	**1275**	

3.8. Reviews and observations

Undertaking correct observations can only carry merit if the frequency of those observations is commensurate with the patient's clinical condition. NCEPOD has alluded to this in a previous report[14]. Of the 885 patients who were deemed to have had appropriate observations 92.8% (570/614) were believed to have had an adequate frequency of those observations (Table 33). (Excluding those 271 cases where there was insufficient data to make a judgement).

Table 33. Was the frequency of clinical observations appropriate?		
	Number of patients	**%**
Yes	570	92.8
No	44	7.2
Subtotal	**614**	
Insufficient data	271	
Total	**885**	

Interestingly, when patients were transferred to an appropriate first ward a similar number received appropriate observations compared with those transferred to an inappropriate first ward. Furthermore, a small number of patients on an appropriate first ward received inappropriate observations compared with a similar number on an inappropriate first ward. While this may provide some reassurance that appropriateness of inpatient ward does not alter appropriateness of observations, it does suggest that across the board appropriateness of observations is lower than expected.

Furthermore, when frequency of observations versus appropriateness of ward was studied, it was of concern that only 63.4% (465/734) of patients received an appropriate frequency of observations despite being on an appropriate ward.

Case study 10 illustrates how inadequate clinical observations can have dire consequences.

Case study 10

An elderly patient was admitted during the daytime on a weekday, via the emergency department, to an emergency assessment unit with a one day history of abdominal pain. The initial assessment, by an SHO, reported a palpable pulsatile abdominal mass. No differential diagnosis was documented. A CT scan was arranged for the next day. The patient was found "cold and stiff" the next morning less than 24 hours after admission.

The advisors were concerned with the quality of documentation received by NCEPOD. It was unclear whether the patient was reviewed by a consultant. Nor did NCEPOD receive any nursing observation charts. The advisors were of the opinion that the fact that the patient was found in rigor mortis suggested the frequency of observations may have been inappropriate. Unfortunately, there was no evidence in the notes that an autopsy was either requested or performed. Did this patient have a leaking abdominal aortic aneurysm that was missed by the admitting doctor?

Key findings

- The level of clinical review of emergency admissions was generally adequate.

- Where the level of clinical review was inadequate this was judged to have affected the diagnosis in 27/76 cases and the outcome in 50/69 cases.

- It was difficult to find clear evidence that emergency admissions received adequate clinical observations, both in type and frequency; moreover there was clear evidence that approximately 6.8% (82/1204) of patients did not.

- Appropriateness of ward did not seem to have an impact on either appropriateness of type of observations or frequency of observations. However, this comment should be interpreted in the context of the denominator representing a large volume of insufficient/blank data.

- Thus it is possible to suggest that not only are appropriate observations performed less often than is desirable, when they are performed, their frequency is inappropriately low in a significant proportion of patients even if they are on a suitable sub-specialty ward.

Recommendations

- All emergency admissions should receive adequate review in line with current national guidance. *(Clinical directors)*

- A clear physiological monitoring plan should be made for each patient commensurate with their clinical condition. This should detail what is to be monitored, the desirable parameters and the frequency of observations. This should be regardless of the type of ward to which the patients are transferred. *(Clinical directors)*

- Part of the treatment plan should be an explicit statement of parameters that should prompt a request for review by medical staff or expert multidisciplinary team (An Acute Problem?). *(Clinical directors)*

3.9. Adverse events

The issue of adverse events is highly topical. The reports "An Organisation with a Memory "[24] and "To Err is human"[25], culminated in the establishment of the National Patient Safety Agency. However, defining and obtaining accurate data regarding adverse events, which are both reliable and valid has proved to be difficult. It is important to understand that the purpose of identifying adverse events in this study was to identify remediable factors in the process of care. It would be inappropriate to draw any conclusions regarding the incidence or range of adverse events occurring in an acute hospital environment given the selective nature of the emergency admission sample in this study.

The Gray report[26] sets out the relationship between adverse events, error and preventability in the Venn diagram in Figure 21.

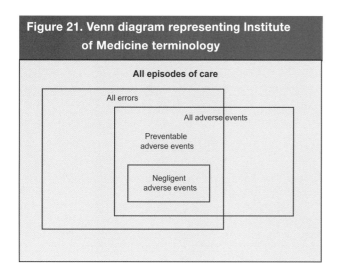

Figure 21. Venn diagram representing Institute of Medicine terminology

All episodes of care

All errors

All adverse events

Preventable adverse events

Negligent adverse events

Ideally, in this study it would have been of benefit if we could have identified those patients who fell into the preventable adverse events group, so that recommendations could be made to improve the quality of care for patients.

In the present study, advisors were asked to assess whether a patient had suffered an adverse event between admission and day 7 of admission. For the purposes of this study, an adverse event was classified, by NCEPOD, as:

"An unintended injury caused by medical management rather than by the disease process and which is sufficiently serious to lead to prolongation of the hospitalisation or to temporary or permanent impairment or disability to the patient at the time of discharge."

Advisors were asked to identify adverse events using this definition.

Initially advisors identified a total of 150 patients who had suffered as a result of an adverse event. However, on further review, only 51 of these cases fulfilled the definition of an adverse event specified above. This in itself gives some idea of the scale of the problem when interpreting the various definitions which exist for adverse incidents.

A total of 51 adverse events were identified out of the 1275 cases which represents a very small proportion of patients. It is recognised that the most common type of adverse event in hospital is associated with the administration of drugs. However it should be noted that although drug charts were requested they were not always supplied; thus a systematic assessment of the true number of adverse events was not possible from this study.

In 14/51 adverse events there was a delay in identifying the event, and in 7/51 cases there was a delay in responding to the event. In 4/7 the delay was attributable to clinical aspects of care, and in 2/7 attributable to organisational aspects, with one case demonstrating delay in both aspects.

Advisors were asked to comment upon the impact of the event upon the patient.

In 16/51 cases there was prolongation of hospitalisation, in three cases there was permanent impairment or disability to the patient at the time of discharge, and in 22 cases, death was thought to have been partly attributable to the adverse event (Table 34).

Table 34. Impact of the event		
	Number of events	%
Prolongation of hospitalisation	16	31.4
Permanent impairment or disability	3	5.9
Death	22	43.1
Insufficient data	10	19.6
Total	51	

Case study 11 is a short example of one such type of adverse event

Case study 11

An alcohol-dependent patient on diazepam, dihydrocodeine, chlormethiazole and other analgesics, was noted to be agitated and recorded as having an oxygen saturation of 91%. Nursing handover was poor, and medical staff appeared to be unaware of the situation. No blood gases were obtained. The patient subsequently died of a cardio-respiratory arrest.

Key finding

- The data provided to NCEPOD, particularly relating to drug administration was incomplete, and therefore it has proved difficult to identify adverse events. Further difficulties arose from the lack of consistency in interpretation of definitions surrounding adverse events.

Recommendation

- Further work is required by the NPSA to educate and inform clinical staff about the definitions surrounding adverse events. There must be standardisation of reporting and audit of that reporting to ensure that accurate data is obtained. (National patient safety agency)

References

1. *Hospital Episode Statistics 2004/5*
   Department of Health.
   http://www.hesonline.nhs.uk

2. *Accident and emergency: Acute Hospital Portfolio.*
   Audit Commission. London 2001.
   http://www.audit-commission.gov.uk/reports/AC-REPORT.asp?CatID=&ProdID=037F9E79-DF51-4823-96B9-E87DF4B58EB9

3. *Bed management: Acute Hospital Portfolio.*
   Audit Commission London. 2003.
   http://www.audit-commission.gov.uk/reports/accessible.asp?ProdID=81EE0CB0-9FED-11d7-B304-0060085F8572

4. *Reforming Emergency Care - Practical Steps.*
   Department of Health. 2004.
   http://www.dh.gov.uk/en/Publicationsandstatistics/Publications/PublicationsPolicyAndGuidance/DH_4092955

5. *Improving the flow of emergency admissions – key questions and steps.*
   Modernisation Agency. 2001.
   http://www.dh.gov.uk/en/Publicationsandstatistics/Publications/PublicationsPolicyAndGuidance/DH_4007914

6. *Ideal Design of Emergency Access (IDEA) Programme.*
   Modernisation Agency. 2002.

7. *Houghton A, Hopkins A. Acute medical admissions: results of a national audit.*
   J R Coll Physicians London 1996;30(6):551-559.

8. *The Society for Acute Medicine, UK.*
   http://www.acutemedicine.org.uk/Guidelines/maguidelines.htm

9. *The interface of Accident and Emergency and Acute Medicine.*
   The Royal College of Physicians of London. 2002.
   http://www.rcplondon.ac.uk/pubs/brochure.aspx?e=110

10. *A guide to Emergency Medical and Surgical Admissions.*
    Department of Health. 2005.
    http://www.dh.gov.uk/en/Publicationsandstatistics/Publications/PublicationsPolicyAndGuidance/DH_4121900

11. *Cooke MW HJ, Kidd P. Use of emergency observation and assessment wards: a systematic literature review.*
    Emerg Med J 2003;20:138-142.

12. *Alberti G. Emergency Assessment Units – a Checklist. 2003.*
    http://www.dh.gov.uk/en/Publicationsandstatistics/Publications/PublicationsPolicyAndGuidance/DH_4010048

13. *Acute medicine, making it work for patients. A report of a working party 2004.*
    The Royal College of Physicians of London.
    http://www.rcplondon.ac.uk/pubs/books/AcuteMedicine/AcuteMedicineFull.pdf

14. *An Acute Problem?*
    National Confidential Enquiry into Patient Outcome and Death. 2005.
    http//www.ncepod.org.uk

15. *Standardisation of clerking proformae*
    Personal Communication.
    The Royal College of Physicians of London. 2007.

16. *Seward E, Greig E, Preston S et al. A confidential study of deaths after emergency medical admission: issues relating to quality of care.*
Clin Med 2003;3:425–34.

17. *Good medical practice for physicians, 2004.*
The Royal College of Physicians of London.
http://www.rcplondon.ac.uk/files/ GoodMedicalPracticeForPhysicians.pdf

18. *Alberti G. Transforming Emergency Care in England 2004.*
http://www.dh.gov.uk/en/Publicationsandstatistics/ Publications/PublicationsPolicyAndGuidance/ DH_4091775

19. *The Emergency Department: Medicine and Surgery Interface Problems and Solutions.*
The Royal College of Surgeons of England. 2004.
http://www.rcseng.ac.uk/rcseng/content/publications/ docs/emergency_department.html

20. *Good surgical practice.*
The Royal College of Surgeons of England. 2002.
http://www.rcseng.ac.uk/publications/docs/good_ surgical_practice.html

21. *Future patterns of care by general and specialist physicians.*
Report of a Working Party.
The Royal College of Physicians of London. 1996.

22. *Acute Medicine Admissions and the Future of General Medicine.*
Report of a Working Party.
The Royal College of Physicians of Edinburgh. 1998.

23. *Black CM. Acute medicine: the physician's future role.*
The Journal of the Royal College of Physicians of London 2000;34(3).

24. *An Organisation with a Memory.*
Department of Health. 2003.
http://www.dh.gov.uk/en/Publicationsandstatistics/ Publications/PublicationsPolicyAndGuidance/ DH_4065083

25 *To Err is human: Building a Safer Health Service.*
Institute of Medicine. 2000.
http://www.nap.edu/books/0309068371/html/

26. *Gray A. Adverse events and the National Health Service an economic perspective.*
A report to the National Patient Safety Agency. 2003.
http://www.npsa.nhs.uk/site/media/documents/941_ AGrayfinalreport1103.pdf

27. *Safer care for the acutely ill patient: learning from critical incidents.*
National Patient Safety Agency. 2007.
http://www.npsa.nhs.uk/site/media/ documents/2840_0559_PSO_Acutely_Ill_Web.pdf

28. *Acutely ill patients in hospital. Recognition of and response to illness in adults in hospital.*
NICE Clinical Guideline 50. National Institute for Health and Clinical Excellence. 2007.
http://guidance.nice.org.uk/CG50

Appendix A – Glossary and abbreviations

AF	Assessment form
AF	Atrial fibrillation
BP	Blood pressure
CT	Computed tomography
EAU	Emergency Assessment Unit
ECG	Electrocardiogram
ED	Emergency department
ENT	Ear, nose and throat
FY2	Foundation year 2
GCS	Glasgow Coma Score/Scale
GI	Gastrointestinal
GP	General practitioner
HES	Hospital episode statistics
ICP	Intracranial pressure

ICU	Intensive care unit
IV	Intravenous
kPa	Kilo Pascals
mmHg	Millimetres of mercury
MRCP(UK)	Membership of the Royal College of Physicians (UK)
NHS	National Health Service
NHSIA	NHS Information Authority
NPSA	National Patient Safety Agency
ONS	Office for National Statistics
PRHO	Pre-registration House Officer
SHO	Senior House Officer
SpR	Specialist Registrar
TPR	Temperature, pulse, respiration

Appendix B – Trust participation

Trust	Cases identified	Cases included	Clinical questionnaires received	Organisational questionnaire/s received
Adur, Arun and Worthing Primary Care Trust	Yes	No	N/A	No
Aintree University Hospitals NHS Foundation Trust	Yes	Yes	Yes	Yes
Airedale NHS Trust	Yes	Yes	Yes	Yes
Ashford & St Peter's Hospital NHS Trust	Yes	Yes	Yes	No
Barking, Havering and Redbridge Hospitals NHS Trust	Yes	Yes	Yes	Yes
Barnet and Chase Farm Hospitals NHS Trust	Yes	Yes	Yes	No
Barnsley Hospital NHS Foundation Trust	Yes	Yes	Yes	Yes
Barnsley Primary Care Trust	Yes	No	N/A	No
Bart's and The London NHS Trust	Yes	Yes	Yes	Yes
Basildon & Thurrock University Hospitals NHS Foundation Trust	Yes	No	N/A	No
Bedford Hospital NHS Trust	Yes	Yes	Yes	Yes
Bedfordshire Heartlands Primary Care Trust	Yes	No	N/A	No
Belfast City Hospital Health & Social Services Trust	Yes	Yes	Yes	Yes
Birmingham Heartlands & Solihull (Teaching) NHS Trust	Yes	Yes	Yes	No
Blackpool, Fylde and Wyre Hospitals NHS Trust	Yes	Yes	Yes	Yes
BMI Healthcare	Yes	No	N/A	No
Bolton Hospitals NHS Trust	Yes	Yes	Yes	Yes
Bradford Teaching Hospitals NHS Foundation Trust	Yes	Yes	Yes	Yes
Brighton and Sussex University Hospitals NHS Trust	Yes	Yes	Yes	Yes
Bro Morgannwg NHS Trust	Yes	Yes	Yes	Yes
Buckinghamshire Hospitals NHS Trust	Yes	Yes	Yes	Yes
BUPA	Yes	No	N/A	No
Burton Hospitals NHS Trust	Yes	Yes	Yes	Yes
Cambridge University Hospitals NHS Foundation Trust	Yes	Yes	Yes	Yes
Capio Health Care UK	Yes	No	N/A	No
Cardiff and Vale NHS Trust	Yes	Yes	Yes	Yes

Appendix B – Trust participation

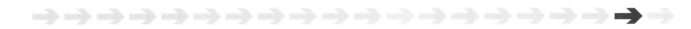

Trust	Cases identified	Cases included	Clinical questionnaires received	Organisational questionnaire/s received
Cardiothoracic Centre Liverpool NHS Trust (The)	Yes	Yes	Yes	Yes
Central Cornwall Primary Care Trust	Yes	No	N/A	No
Central Manchester & Manchester Children's University Hospitals NHS Trust	Yes	Yes	Yes	Yes
Chelsea & Westminster Healthcare NHS Trust	Yes	Yes	Yes	Yes
Chesterfield & North Derbyshire Royal Hospital NHS Trust	Yes	Yes	Yes	Yes
Chorley and South Ribble Primary Care Trust	Yes	Yes	Yes	Yes
Christie Hospital NHS Trust	Yes	No	N/A	No
City Hospitals Sunderland NHS Foundation Trust	Yes	Yes	Yes	Yes
Clatterbridge Centre for Oncology NHS Trust	Yes	No	N/A	No
Conwy & Denbighshire NHS Trust	Yes	Yes	Yes	Yes
Countess of Chester Hospital NHS Foundation Trust	Yes	No	N/A	No
County Durham and Darlington Acute Hospitals NHS Trust	Yes	Yes	Yes	Yes
Craigavon Area Hospital Group Trust	Yes	Yes	Yes	Yes
Cromwell Hospital	Yes	No	N/A	No
Dartford & Gravesham NHS Trust	Yes	Yes	Yes	Yes
Derby Hospitals NHS Foundation Trust	Yes	Yes	Yes	Yes
Doncaster and Bassetlaw Hospitals NHS Foundation Trust	Yes	Yes	Yes	Yes
Down Lisburn Health & Social Services Trust	Yes	Yes	Yes	No
Dudley Group of Hospitals NHS Trust	Yes	Yes	Yes	Yes
Ealing Hospital NHS Trust	Yes	Yes	Yes	No
East Cheshire NHS Trust	Yes	Yes	Yes	Yes
East Kent Hospitals NHS Trust	Yes	Yes	Yes	Yes
East Lancashire Hospitals NHS Trust	Yes	Yes	Yes	Yes
East Somerset NHS Trust	Yes	Yes	Yes	Yes
East Sussex Hospitals NHS Trust	Yes	Yes	Yes	Yes

Trust	Cases identified	Cases included	Clinical questionnaires received	Organisational questionnaire/s received
Epsom and St Helier University Hospitals NHS Trust	Yes	Yes	Yes	Yes
Essex Rivers Healthcare NHS Trust	Yes	Yes	Yes	Yes
Frimley Park Hospitals NHS Trust	Yes	Yes	Yes	No
George Eliot Hospital NHS Trust	Yes	Yes	Yes	Yes
Good Hope Hospital NHS Trust	Yes	Yes	Yes	Yes
Guy's & St Thomas' Hospital NHS Foundation Trust	Yes	Yes	Yes	No
Gwent Healthcare NHS Trust	Yes	Yes	Yes	Yes
Hammersmith Hospitals NHS Trust	Yes	Yes	Yes	Yes
Harrogate and District NHS Foundation Trust	Yes	Yes	Yes	Yes
Harrow Primary Care Trust	Yes	Yes	No	No
HCA International	Yes	Yes	Yes	Yes
Heatherwood and Wexham Park Hospitals NHS Trust	Yes	Yes	Yes	Yes
Hereford Hospitals NHS Trust	Yes	Yes	Yes	Yes
Hinchingbrooke Health Care NHS Trust	Yes	Yes	Yes	Yes
Homerton University Hospital NHS Foundation Trust	Yes	Yes	Yes	Yes
Hull and East Yorkshire Hospitals NHS Trust	Yes	Yes	Yes	Yes
Ipswich Hospital NHS Trust	Yes	Yes	Yes	Yes
Isle of Man Department of Health & Social Security	Yes	Yes	Yes	Yes
Isle of Wight Healthcare NHS Trust	Yes	Yes	Yes	Yes
James Paget Healthcare NHS Trust	Yes	Yes	Yes	Yes
Kennet and North Wiltshire Primary Care Trust	Yes	Yes	Yes	No
Kettering General Hospital NHS Trust	Yes	Yes	Yes	Yes
King's College Hospital NHS Trust	Yes	Yes	Yes	Yes
King's Lynn & Wisbech Hospitals NHS Trust	Yes	Yes	Yes	Yes
Kingston Hospital NHS Trust	Yes	Yes	Yes	Yes
Lancashire Teaching Hospitals NHS Trust	Yes	No	N/A	Yes
Leeds Teaching Hospitals NHS Trust (The)	Yes	Yes	Yes	Yes

Appendix B – Trust participation

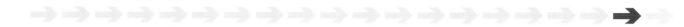

Trust	Cases identified	Cases included	Clinical questionnaires received	Organisational questionnaire/s received
London Clinic	Yes	No	N/A	No
Luton and Dunstable Hospital NHS Trust	Yes	Yes	Yes	Yes
Maidstone and Tunbridge Wells NHS Trust	Yes	Yes	Yes	No
Maldon & South Chelmsford PCT	Yes	No	N/A	No
Mater Hospital Belfast Health & Social Services Trust	Yes	No	N/A	No
Mayday Health Care NHS Trust	Yes	Yes	Yes	No
Medway NHS Trust	Yes	Yes	Yes	No
Mid Cheshire Hospitals NHS Trust	Yes	Yes	No	Yes
Mid Staffordshire General Hospitals NHS Trust	Yes	Yes	Yes	Yes
Mid Yorkshire Hospitals NHS Trust	Yes	Yes	Yes	Yes
Mid-Essex Hospital Services NHS Trust	Yes	Yes	Yes	No
Moorfields Eye Hospital NHS Foundation Trust	Yes	No	N/A	No
Morecambe Bay Hospitals NHS Trust	Yes	Yes	Yes	Yes
Newcastle upon Tyne Hospitals NHS Trust	Yes	Yes	Yes	Yes
Newham Healthcare NHS Trust	Yes	Yes	Yes	Yes
Norfolk & Norwich University Hospital NHS Trust	Yes	Yes	Yes	Yes
North Bristol NHS Trust	Yes	Yes	Yes	Yes
North Cheshire Hospitals NHS Trust	Yes	Yes	Yes	Yes
North Cumbria Acute Hospitals NHS Trust	Yes	Yes	Yes	No
North Devon Primary Care Trust	Yes	Yes	Yes	No
North East Wales NHS Trust	Yes	Yes	Yes	Yes
North Glamorgan NHS Trust	Yes	Yes	Yes	Yes
North Hampshire Hospitals NHS Trust	Yes	Yes	Yes	No
North Middlesex University Hospital NHS Trust	Yes	Yes	Yes	No
North Tees and Hartlepool NHS Trust	Yes	Yes	Yes	Yes
North West London Hospitals NHS Trust	Yes	Yes	Yes	Yes
Northampton General Hospital NHS Trust	Yes	Yes	Yes	Yes
Northern Devon Healthcare NHS Trust	Yes	Yes	Yes	No

Trust	Cases identified	Cases included	Clinical questionnaires received	Organisational questionnaire/s received
Northern Lincolnshire & Goole Hospitals Trust	Yes	Yes	Yes	Yes
Northumbria Healthcare NHS Trust	Yes	Yes	Yes	Yes
Nottingham City Hospital NHS Trust	Yes	Yes	Yes	Yes
Nuffield	Yes	No	N/A	No
Nuffield Orthopaedic Centre NHS Trust	Yes	No	N/A	No
Oxford Radcliffe Hospital NHS Trust	Yes	Yes	Yes	Yes
Pennine Acute Hospitals NHS Trust (The)	Yes	Yes	Yes	Yes
Peterborough & Stamford Hospitals NHS FoundationTrust	Yes	Yes	Yes	Yes
Plymouth Hospitals NHS Trust	Yes	Yes	Yes	Yes
Plymouth Primary Care Trust	Yes	No	N/A	No
Pontypridd & Rhondda NHS Trust	Yes	Yes	Yes	Yes
Poole Hospital NHS Trust	Yes	Yes	Yes	No
Portsmouth Hospitals NHS Trust	Yes	Yes	Yes	No
Princess Alexandra Hospital NHS Trust	Yes	Yes	Yes	Yes
Queen Elizabeth Hospital NHS Trust	Yes	Yes	Yes	Yes
Queen Mary's Sidcup NHS Trust	Yes	Yes	Yes	Yes
Queen Victoria Hospital NHS Foundation Trust	Yes	No	N/A	No
Queen's Medical Centre Nottingham University Hospital NHS Trust	Yes	Yes	Yes	Yes
Robert Jones and Agnes Hunt Orthopaedic and District Hospital NHS Trust	Yes	No	N/A	No
Rotherham General Hospitals NHS Trust	Yes	Yes	Yes	Yes
Royal Berkshire and Battle Hospitals NHS Trust	Yes	Yes	Yes	Yes
Royal Bournemouth and Christchurch Hospitals NHS Trust	Yes	Yes	Yes	Yes
Royal Brompton and Harefield NHS Trust	Yes	Yes	Yes	Yes
Royal Cornwall Hospitals NHS Trust	Yes	Yes	Yes	Yes
Royal Devon and Exeter NHS Foundation Trust	Yes	Yes	Yes	Yes
Royal Free Hampstead NHS Trust	Yes	Yes	Yes	Yes

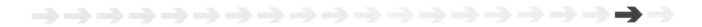

Trust	Cases identified	Cases included	Clinical questionnaires received	Organisational questionnaire/s received
Royal Group of Hospitals & Dental Hospitals & Maternity Hospitals Trust	Yes	Yes	Yes	Yes
Royal Liverpool and Broadgreen University Hospitals NHS Trust	Yes	Yes	Yes	Yes
Royal Liverpool Children's NHS Trust	Yes	No	N/A	No
Royal Marsden NHS Foundation Trust (The)	Yes	Yes	Yes	No
Royal United Hospital Bath NHS Trust	Yes	Yes	Yes	Yes
Royal West Sussex NHS Trust	Yes	Yes	Yes	Yes
Royal Wolverhampton Hospitals NHS Trust (The)	Yes	Yes	Yes	Yes
Salford Royal Hospitals NHS Trust	Yes	Yes	Yes	Yes
Salisbury Health Care NHS Trust	Yes	Yes	Yes	Yes
Sandwell and West Birmingham Hospitals NHS Trust	Yes	Yes	Yes	Yes
Scarborough and North East Yorkshire Health Care NHS Trust	Yes	Yes	Yes	Yes
Sheffield Teaching Hospitals NHS Foundation Trust	Yes	Yes	Yes	Yes
Sherwood Forest Hospitals NHS Trust	Yes	Yes	Yes	No
Shrewsbury and Telford Hospitals NHS Trust	Yes	Yes	Yes	Yes
Shropshire County Primary Care Trust	Yes	Yes	No	No
South Devon Healthcare NHS Trust	Yes	Yes	Yes	Yes
South Manchester University Hospitals NHS Trust	Yes	Yes	Yes	Yes
South Tees Hospitals NHS Trust	Yes	Yes	Yes	Yes
South Tyneside Healthcare Trust	Yes	Yes	Yes	Yes
South Warwickshire General Hospitals NHS Trust	Yes	Yes	Yes	Yes
Southampton University Hospitals NHS Trust	Yes	Yes	Yes	Yes
Southport and Ormskirk Hospitals NHS Trust	Yes	Yes	Yes	Yes
St Anthony's Hospital	Yes	Yes	No	No
St George's Healthcare NHS Trust	Yes	Yes	Yes	Yes
St Helens and Knowsley Hospitals NHS Trust	Yes	Yes	Yes	Yes
St Mary's NHS Trust	Yes	Yes	Yes	Yes

Trust	Cases identified	Cases included	Clinical questionnaires received	Organisational questionnaire/s received
States of Guernsey Board of Health	Yes	Yes	Yes	Yes
Stockport NHS Foundation Trust	Yes	Yes	Yes	Yes
Surrey & Sussex Healthcare NHS Trust	Yes	Yes	Yes	Yes
Swansea NHS Trust	Yes	Yes	Yes	Yes
Swindon & Marlborough NHS Trust	Yes	Yes	Yes	Yes
Tameside and Glossop Acute Services NHS Trust	Yes	Yes	Yes	Yes
Taunton & Somerset NHS Trust	Yes	Yes	Yes	Yes
Trafford Healthcare NHS Trust	Yes	Yes	Yes	Yes
Ulster Community & Hospitals NHS Trust	Yes	Yes	No	Yes
United Bristol Healthcare NHS Trust	Yes	Yes	Yes	Yes
United Hospitals Health & Social Services Trust	Yes	Yes	Yes	Yes
United Lincolnshire Hospitals NHS Trust	Yes	Yes	Yes	Yes
University College London Hospitals NHS Foundation Trust	Yes	Yes	Yes	No
University Hospital Birmingham NHS Foundation Trust	Yes	Yes	Yes	Yes
University Hospital of North Staffordshire NHS Trust	Yes	Yes	Yes	Yes
University Hospitals Coventry and Warwickshire NHS Trust	Yes	Yes	Yes	Yes
University Hospitals of Leicester NHS Trust	Yes	Yes	Yes	Yes
Walsall Hospitals NHS Trust	Yes	Yes	Yes	No
Waveney Primary Care Trust	Yes	Yes	No	Yes
West Dorset General Hospitals NHS Trust	Yes	Yes	Yes	Yes
West Hertfordshire Hospitals NHS Trust	Yes	Yes	Yes	No
West Middlesex University Hospital NHS Trust	Yes	Yes	Yes	No
West Suffolk Hospitals NHS Trust	Yes	Yes	Yes	Yes
West Wiltshire Primary Care Trust	Yes	No	N/A	No
Weston Area Health Trust	Yes	Yes	Yes	No
Whipps Cross University Hospital NHS Trust	Yes	Yes	Yes	Yes
Whittington Hospital NHS Trust	Yes	Yes	Yes	No

Appendix B – Trust participation

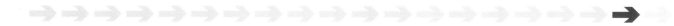

Trust	Cases identified	Cases included	Clinical questionnaires received	Organisational questionnaire/s received
Winchester & Eastleigh Healthcare NHS Trust	Yes	Yes	Yes	Yes
Wirral Hospital NHS Trust	Yes	Yes	Yes	No
Witham, Baintree & Halstead Care Trust	Yes	No	N/A	No
Worcestershire Acute Hospitals	Yes	Yes	Yes	No
Worthing and Southlands Hospitals NHS Trust	Yes	Yes	Yes	Yes
Wrightington, Wigan & Leigh NHS Trust	Yes	Yes	Yes	Yes
York Hospitals NHS Trust	Yes	Yes	Yes	No

NB: Trusts not listed did not identify cases for the study, this may have been because there were no suitable cases during the study period or the trust did not accept emergency admissions. Trust names are listed as at the time of data collection not publication.

Appendix C – Corporate structure

The National Confidential Enquiry into Patient Outcome and Death (NCEPOD) is an independent body to which a corporate commitment has been made by the Medical and Surgical Colleges, Associations and Faculties related to its area of activity. Each of these bodies nominates members on to NCEPOD's Steering Group

Steering Group as at 10th October 2007

Dr D Whitaker
Association of Anaesthetists of Great Britain and Ireland

Mr T Bates
Association of Surgeons of Great Britain & Ireland

Dr S Bridgman
Faculty of Public Health Medicine

Dr P Cartwright
Royal College of Anaesthetists

Dr P Nightingale
Royal College of Anaesthetists

Dr B Ellis
Royal College of General Practitioners

Ms M McElligott
Royal College of Nursing

Prof D Luesley
Royal College of Obstetricians and Gynaecologists

Mrs M Wishart
Royal College of Ophthalmologists

Dr I Doughty
Royal College of Paediatrics and Child Health

Dr R Dowdle
Royal College of Physicians

Professor T Hendra
Royal College of Physicians

Dr M Armitage
Royal College of Physicians

Dr M Clements
Royal College of Physicians

Dr A Nicholson
Royal College of Radiologists

Mr B Rees
Royal College of Surgeons of England

Mr D Mitchell
*Faculty of Dental Surgery,
Royal College of Surgeons of England*

Dr S Lishman
Royal College of Pathologists

Ms S Panizzo
Patient Representative

Mrs M Wang
Patient Representative